RUNNER'S WORLD
PERFORMANCE
NUTRITION
FOR RUNNERS

RUNNER'S **WORLD**®

PERFORMANCE NUTRITION
FOR RUNNERS

HOW TO FUEL YOUR BODY FOR STRONGER
WORKOUTS, FASTER RECOVERY,
AND YOUR BEST RACE TIMES EVER

MATT FITZGERALD

RODALE

Photographs by Mitch Mandel
Book design by Anthony Serge

Library of Congress Cataloging-in-Publication Data

Fitzgerald, Matt.
    Runner's world performance nutrition for runners : how to fuel your body for stronger workouts, faster recovery, and your best race times ever / Matt Fitzgerald.
        p.   cm.
    Includes index.
    ISBN-13 978–1–59486–218–2 paperback
    ISBN-10 1–59486–218–4 paperback
    1. Runners (Sports)—Nutrition.   2. Athletes—Nutrition.   I. Title.
TX361.R86F58   2006
613'.02479642—dc22   2005026758

Distributed to the trade by Holtzbrinck Publishers

    4   6   8   10   9   7   5   3   paperback

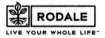

FOR MY BROTHERS, JOSH AND SEAN

CONTENTS

ACKNOWLEDGMENTS

I would like to express my deepest gratitude to the many people whose help and support made this book possible and better than it otherwise would have been. Most especially, I wish to thank Lawrence Armstrong, Rich Benyo, Dan Browne, Leah Flickinger, Jeff Galloway, Christina Gandolfo, Paul Goldberg, Jane Hahn, Kim Mueller-Brown, John Ivy, Deena Kastor, Tim Noakes, Andrea Pedolsky, Robert Portman, Lonna Ramirez, Evelyn Tribole, Alan Webb, Walter Willett, and my family.

INTRODUCTION

Nutrition is vitally important in every sport. The right nutrition provides a host of benefits from enhanced workout performance to reduced injury risk. Nutrition errors, on the other hand, can hold you back by compromising post-workout recovery, for example, or causing your muscles to fatigue prematurely.

Some nutrition guidelines apply to all athletes. Every athlete is human, after all, and each human being shares the same basic nutrition needs. But runners have their own special nutrition requirements. For example, hydration and energy consumption during training and competition are more important to runners than to most other athletes, because they sweat more and burn more calories than many other types of athletes. At the same time, fueling on the run is more challenging than fueling in most other sports, because most runners don't want to slow down or stop to drink (at least during races) and because the stomach jostling involved in running makes it hard to tolerate a high stomach volume. So runners require innovative approaches to fueling their bodies. Running also results in a tremendous amount of muscle tissue damage compared to other sports. The right nutrition practices will reduce the amount of running-related muscle damage you experience and will accelerate the muscle repair process. Similar practices may also benefit athletes in other sports, but for runners the cost of not using them is far greater.

Body weight is another special concern for runners. A low body weight is more beneficial in running than in many other sports, as every ounce adds to the load your muscles have to lift and push forward with each stride. Yet runners must be very careful how they seek to achieve their best "race weight." Severe calorie restriction (dieting) is likely to shed some pounds, but it is also likely to increase your risk of injury and to ruin your workouts by sapping your energy stores. Runners need a more sophisticated approach than dieting to achieve their best race weight.

There are many general nutrition resources for athletes, and even several for endurance athletes, but very few that address the nutrition requirements and challenges of runners only. Using the very latest sports and nutrition science and my more than 20 years of personal experience as a runner and running coach, I wrote this book to satisfy the glaring need for such a resource.

In the following chapters, you will learn everything you need to know to enhance your running performance with nutrition. This includes information on using nutrition to boost your overall health, because anything that benefits your health benefits your running as well. I will share cutting-edge strategies for how to fuel your body for maximum performance in workouts and races, how to optimize your body composition, how to minimize running-related muscle damage, and dozens of other tips to help you get the most out of your running.

Your training is already customized to your needs and goals as a runner. Get ready to take your nutrition to the same level—and to achieve maximum performance as a result.

CHAPTER 1
WHAT IS PERFORMANCE NUTRITION?

Doping in sports has been big news in recent years. The use of illegal performance-enhancing drugs and of other banned measures such as blood doping has reached crisis proportions. While the sports of baseball, football, cycling, and track & field have been hit the hardest, long-distance running has been hit, too.

One of the most dramatic blows fell in 2000, when former 5000-meter world record holder Dong Yanmei and six other Chinese runners were cut from the Chinese Olympic Team after testing positive for use of synthetic EPO (short for erythropoietin, a blood-boosting hormone). The following year, closer to home, Regina Jacobs, the 5000-meter American record holder, tested positive for the synthetic steroid THG. And the year after that, Brahim Boulami of Morocco, world record holder in the 3000-meter steeplechase, was banned from the sport for 2 years for using EPO.

In this same period of time, I became involved in an advocacy group called Powering Muscles that sought to address the problem of doping in sports. An initiative of the United States Track Coaches

Association, Powering Muscles was a multidisciplinary educational effort involving exercise physiologists, nutritionists, track coaches, and athletes that was designed to teach other track coaches, trainers, and athletes about the role of nutrition in athletic performance. Our overarching goal was to reduce athletes' use of performance-enhancing drugs by demonstrating that nutrition offers a safer and equally effective alternative.

Most runners believe (or at least assume) that no legitimate alternative can match the performance-boosting effects of a drug such as EPO. It's probably true that no *single* legitimate alternative to doping can do so, but I and many other experts strongly believe that a runner who takes full advantage of *every* legitimate means to enhance performance can reach the same performance level that he or she would reach through the shortcut of doping (not to mention sustain it longer and do it without ruining his or her long-term health). In addition to cutting-edge nutritional practices, effective alternatives to cheating may include sleeping in an altitude simulation tent, cross-training, better mental preparation, running technique improvement, and state-of-the-art injury avoidance and treatment measures.

It's difficult to overstate the performance-enhancing potential of natural foods and dietary supplements. In fact, proper nutrition is itself an important facet of training effectively, preventing injuries, and almost everything else you do as a runner. Imagine you have an identical twin, also a runner, with whom you train every day. The only difference between the two of you is that your diet and sports nutrition habits are careless, whereas your twin's diet and sports nutrition habits are based on sound principles and the latest knowledge. Who will have better results? Science tells us your twin will perform better in workouts, recover faster from workouts, gain fitness faster, develop a leaner body composition, be able to handle a heavier training load, get sick less often, suffer fewer injuries, and, most of all, kick your butt in races! And if you don't wise up and start eating and drinking as your twin does, he or she will continue running strong long after age slows you down and will even outlive you. That's how important it is to learn how to fuel your body properly.

I use the term "performance nutrition" with deliberate awareness of the way it echoes "performance-enhancing drugs," because I want runners to understand that it is just as powerful. Performance nutrition is simply a systematic approach to using food and nutritional supplements to enhance running performance. There are six specific objectives of using nutrition in this way, what I call the Six Pillars of Performance Nutrition:

1. Enhance your general health
2. Maximize your body's adaptations to training
3. Fuel running performance
4. Enhance post-exercise recovery
5. Prevent injuries and sickness
6. "Improve on nature"

In this chapter, I will speak generally about these six components of performance nutrition for runners. In the context of these explanations, I will also introduce to you some of the key nutrients, terms, and concepts that will come up again in later chapters, which are entirely devoted to delivering practical strategies to achieve optimal performance nutrition.

USING NUTRITION TO ENHANCE YOUR GENERAL HEALTH

Running fitness and general health are not identical, but they overlap substantially. For example, running fitness depends in part on having a strong heart and excellent blood circulation. These same attributes are also associated with longevity, as they reduce the risk of common causes of death such as stroke and heart attack. Running fitness also depends on having a lean body composition (low body fat percentage), which in addition to helping you run well reduces your risk of diabetes, Alzheimer's, and other diseases.

Because there is so much overlap between running fitness and general health, virtually every factor that has a positive effect on your health is likely to have a positive effect on your running fitness. Examples of such factors are getting adequate sleep and practicing effective stress management. Another one is, of course, nutrition. Maintaining a healthy diet will enhance your overall health in a variety of ways, and a majority of these positive health effects will carry over into your running.

Let's consider aging. One well-known cause of aging is damage to body tissues caused by free radicals, mainly oxygen radicals, which are produced as a normal by-product of aerobic metabolism. Oxygen radicals are missing one electron, making them highly unstable and causing them to steal electrons from healthy tissues. This process can instigate a chain reaction of damage to cell membranes, DNA, and other body proteins. The body uses antioxidant defenses—including enzymes such as superoxide dismutase and nutrients like vitamin E— to prevent and limit free radical damage, but in the long run it's a losing battle. The accumulation of such damage leads to declining function in every organ and system of the body. It is also implicated in the development of a variety of degenerative diseases, including cancers and coronary heart disease.

Good nutrition can bolster antioxidant defenses and thereby slow the aging process. Recent research on simple organisms has shown that increasing the concentration of key antioxidants through genetic manipulation and other means can drastically increase life span. Numerous studies with humans have demonstrated that diets rich in antioxidants such as vitamins C and E and carotenoids reduce the risk and in some cases slow the progression of cancers, Alzheimer's disease, and other degenerative diseases.

The accumulation of free radical damage to body tissues that comes with aging is also one of the primary reasons our running performance declines as we age. As consequences of this damage, our muscles become weaker and less elastic, our heart muscle loses power, and so forth. Good nutrition helps us better maintain our running performance over the years—not to mention enhances it at any age, including in the very prime of life—by strengthening the body's antioxidant defenses. Exercise itself strengthens the body's antioxidant defenses, slowing the aging process and boosting our ability to resist muscle damage during exercise and recover quickly between runs. But the size of this boost depends on how well it is supported by the right nutrition. Consistent training and good nutrition therefore work synergistically to keep us young and swift.

So how exactly do you eat to maximize your general health? In the following chapter, I will identify four simple rules of healthy eating and show you how to follow them.

USING NUTRITION TO MAXIMIZE TRAINING

Running fitness is not a single thing but is rather a collection of interrelated physiological changes in the body that occur in response to training. Individual workouts challenge the functional limitations of our organs and systems (the cardiovascular system, the endocrine system, and so forth). Such stress signals the genes that regulate the affected organs and systems to respond by producing more of certain proteins and less of others—whatever it takes to make the organ or system in question better able to handle the stress of the next workout. The sum of these changes is steadily improving running fitness:

the ability to run faster, farther, more efficiently, and with less chance of injury.

The itemized list of adaptations that occur in the body in response to training is long—and getting longer as exercise scientists continue to explore deeper into the frontier of the human body at work. While exercise stimulates these adaptations, it is the nutrients in your diet that produce them. In other words, exercise only creates a demand in your body for the nutrients that are needed to make fitness-boosting changes. It is nutrition that fulfills this demand. Following are examples of important fitness adaptations that occur in several areas of the body in response to a consistent, progressive running program complemented by an appropriate dietary regimen.

REDUCED BODY FAT

To be healthy, the average human male must have a minimum of 5 percent body fat and the average female must have a minimum of 10 percent body fat. Carrying too little body fat can cause a variety of serious health problems, including immune system depression and reproductive disorders. On the other hand, carrying much more than the minimum amount of body fat required for health has disadvantages in terms of running performance because it adds to the load that the muscles must transport. In one study, the addition of 1 kilogram (2.2 pounds) of weight was shown to increase the energy cost of running by 3.5 percent. This loss of economy would turn a 40-minute 10K runner into a 41:28 10K runner. While body fat is not exactly "dead weight"—as it provides a source of energy during low- to moderate-intensity running—even the leanest healthy runners have enough body fat to provide far more energy than they could ever use in a single run.

Training improves body composition by reducing body fat content while preserving muscle. Body fat tends to decrease when more calories are burned than consumed day after day. When a caloric deficit is achieved without exercise, both muscle and body fat are lost. When it is achieved with exercise, more fat and little to no muscle are lost, because exercise creates a demand for muscle tissue, so that more of the calories consumed are used to rebuild and maintain muscle tissue than to replace burned body fat.

ENHANCED BLOODFLOW

The most important job of the blood during running is to transport oxygen to your muscles (including your heart). The more oxygen your blood is able to deliver, the longer you will be able to sustain faster running speeds. Training results in some important blood changes that enhance its ability to deliver oxygen.

Training increases blood volume by as much as 10 percent. It also increases the number of oxygen-carrying proteins attached to red blood cells. Even the dilating capacity of the blood vessels increases as you become fitter. Wider blood vessels allow greater bloodflow.

Nutrients participate in all of these adaptations. A good example is iron, a trace mineral (i.e., a mineral needed in very small amounts) that is necessary for the formation of hemoglobin, a protein that binds oxygen molecules to red blood cells, and myoglobin, a similar protein that transports oxygen into the muscle cells. Training increases the concentration of iron-storing proteins in the body. Consequently, it also increases the number of hemoglobin molecules per red blood cell, as well as the concentration of myoglobin.

STRONGER BONES

Perhaps the most important early adaptation to running is improvement in the capacity of the bones of the lower extremities to absorb ground impact forces without breaking down. When subjected to a regular schedule of repetitive impact forces, the bones of the lower extremities remodel their structure to become stronger and denser.

This remodeling process is essentially a healing response to impact trauma, which works out for the best as long as running volume is increased very gradually and adequate recovery time is always allowed. If the bones are subjected to too much stress too soon, damage will outpace remodeling and a bone strain will result. Bone strains in the tibia (the smaller of the two shin bones) are the most common injury in beginning runners. A severe bone strain can develop into a stress fracture.

Various nutrients play important roles in the impact-related adaptations of bones. The primary components of bone tissue are collagen (a protein) and the minerals calcium and phosphate.

INCREASED BRAINPOWER

Contrary to what you might assume, the brain contributes more to running performance than any other part of the body. First of all, the "program" for the action of running is stored in your brain (like software in a computer), and the more you run, the more this pattern is refined to become increasingly efficient, so you can run at faster speeds with less energy.

Fatigue is also controlled by the brain. While you run, your brain constantly monitors feedback from your body—the temperature of your muscles, the amount of glucose in your bloodstream, the amount of oxygen reaching your heart—to determine whether your health is in any danger. When your brain decides that you may be running yourself into harm's way, it will cut back on the electrical signals it sends to your muscles, forcing you to slow down. It is this "voluntary" slowdown rather than events in your muscles themselves that constitutes fatigue.

The brain is certainly the most adaptable organ in the body. In fact, it is the only organ that adapts to running *while* you're running. Everything else adapts during the recovery periods between workouts. Nutrition affects the performance of the brain during exercise in a variety of ways. For example, consuming carbohydrate during exercise signals your brain that it is safe to send stronger electrical signals to your muscles, allowing you to run harder, because there's an extra fuel supply to supplement what's already stored in your body.

STRONGER HEART

The heart muscle becomes much larger and more powerful in response to training. This allows it to pump a lot more blood per contraction, substantially increasing the maximum rate of oxygen supply to the muscles. Research has shown that the heart stroke volume (i.e., the amount of blood pumped per contraction) of elite runners is often twice that of sedentary individuals. As with all muscles, proteins are the primary structural ingredients of the heart, so its growth involves the accretion of many new proteins in this vital organ.

MORE EFFICIENT MUSCLES

Skeletal muscles adapt to training in literally dozens of known ways, and probably in dozens more ways that are yet to be discovered or fully understood. I'll highlight a few of these changes.

The muscles adapt to impact forces through an injury-response mechanism similar to that of the bones. Various muscles, especially the calves and quadriceps, help the body absorb impact forces by contracting eccentrically—that is, by resisting their own lengthening. Because eccentric contractions essentially pull muscles in two directions simultaneously, they often damage individual muscle fibers. The damaged tissues respond, over time, by remodeling themselves in such a way as to become more resistant to eccentric rupturing.

Running also stimulates big gains in the muscles' capacity to extract oxygen from the bloodstream and use it to metabolize fats, carbohydrate, and to a lesser extent, amino acids for energy. This process depends on capillaries, which are tiny blood vessels that carry oxygen into muscle cells; myoglobin, a protein that transports oxygen molecules within muscle cells; mitochondria, which are the intracellular sites where oxygen is used to break down fats and carbohydrates; and mitochondrial enzymes, which allow this process to take place extremely fast. Training increases the density of capillaries in the muscles, their myoglobin concentration, the number of mitochondria within the muscle cells, and the concentration of mitochondrial enzymes. In addition, it increases glucose and fatty acid transporters in the muscle cell membranes, which in turn increases the efficiency with which the muscle cells can draw carbohydrate and fat fuel from the blood.

Another important muscular adaptation is improved carbohydrate storage. In longer runs, depletion of carbohydrate fuel stores can be a major contributor to fatigue and exhaustion. Most often the problem is depletion of glycogen stores in the leg muscles, but sometimes hypoglycemia—that is, low blood glucose—occurs first. Hypoglycemia results when glycogen is depleted from the liver, as the liver is responsible for regulating blood glucose levels by breaking down glycogen into glucose and releasing it into the bloodstream as necessary.

The carbohydrate storage capacity of the human body is small. The average adult stores about 500 grams of glycogen (400 grams in the muscles and another 100 grams in the liver), as compared to 12 to 18 kilograms of fat. Training can greatly increase the body's glycogen storage capacity. The leg muscles of an elite runner may contain three times as much glycogen as the legs of a sedentary adult. This adaptation allows the well-trained runner to run a heck of a lot farther at relatively high speeds.

Clearly, nutrition plays a significant role in this adaptation, because all of the body's stored glycogen comes from dietary sugars and starches. Also, runners can effectively increase their carbohydrate stores by consuming a sports drink or gel while running. I'll discuss this topic in depth in Chapter 5.

USING NUTRITION TO FUEL RUNNING PERFORMANCE

The expression "You are what you eat" effectively conveys the idea that the nutrients in our diet become the tissues and organs of our bodies. What it fails to convey is the fact that a number of nutrients play active roles during exercise. In other words, you also *do* what you eat.

Following are descriptions of 10 such nutrients and their running-specific roles. There is more detail in these descriptions than you need to commit to memory, but I include it nonetheless for two reasons: first, because these important nutrients will come up again in later chapters; and second, in case you are as fascinated by the workings of the human body as I am.

Branched-chain amino acids. Amino acids are best known as the building blocks of proteins, but they also function in their free form in the body. There are 20 amino acids, three of which—leucine, isoleucine, and valine—are referred to as branched-chain amino acids because of their structure. Unlike other amino acids, branched-chain amino acids can be directly oxidized for energy within muscle cells rather than having to be converted first to glucose in the liver. The muscles initially rely only minimally on branched-chain amino acids during running, but this reliance becomes greater in the later stages of long runs, when the muscles' preferred energy source—glycogen (the storage form of glucose)—runs low. Training enhances the body's capacity to release energy from amino acids during running. This adaptation results in greater endurance.

Calcium. When we think of calcium, we usually think of bones. It's true that 99 percent of the calcium in the human body is contained in bones as calcium phosphate. But calcium also plays a critical role in muscle action. Positively charged calcium ions located at the neuro-muscular junction (the point where nerves attach to muscles) are needed to turn an electrical impulse from the brain into a chemical action causing muscle fibers to contract and relax. Diminishing calcium stores at the neuromuscular junction are closely associated with muscle fatigue.

Fats. Most of the fats, or fatty acids, in the body are stored as tri-glycerides in adipose tissue deposits (fat layers beneath the skin) throughout the body. Even in very lean runners these energy stores are vast compared to carbohydrate stores (mainly glycogen in the muscles and liver), but they are not as easy to access, which is one reason fats are not the muscles' preferred energy source during intense exercise. In order for the body to use them, triglycerides must be converted to free fatty acids and transported to the muscles through the blood-stream, whereas glycogen is available within the muscle cells.

Scientists often measure exercise intensity as a percentage of VO_2max, where 100 percent VO_2max is the maximum rate at which a given athlete's body is able to consume oxygen. At 40 percent VO_2max (an easy jog), fats supply about 50 percent of muscle energy in a typical trained runner. At 80 percent VO_2max (a comfortably brisk run), fats supply only 5 percent of muscle energy. But runners vary widely in their reliance on fat. Some are "natural fat burners" who use more fat and less carbohydrate at any running intensity. Such runners are best suited to racing at longer distances because they are able to conserve their glycogen stores longer.

A small amount of triglycerides are stored within the muscles. These fats are more accessible than adipose triglycerides and are probably the only fats used for muscle energy above 95 percent VO_2max. Training enhances the body's capacity to deliver free fatty acids to the muscles and to oxidize fats within muscle cells.

Glucose/glycogen. Glucose and chains of glucose molecules called glycogen are the primary sources of muscle energy during moderately high- to high-intensity running. They provide virtually all of the energy for sustained running above 95 percent VO_2 max in most runners (except during all-out sprinting, when creatine phosphate is used). Glucose and glycogen are derived from sugars (including glucose itself) and starches consumed in the diet. Training increases the body's capacity to store glycogen in the muscles and liver and to burn glucose and glycogen efficiently. It also enhances the ability of the liver to convert lactate, a product of incomplete glucose metabolism, and amino acids to glucose.

Glutamine. Glutamine is the most abundant amino acid in the blood and skeletal muscles. Most of the body's glutamine is in fact produced by the muscles. It is an important fuel for many cells of the immune system. During running, glutamine also provides an additional source of glucose to fuel muscle contractions. It is sent from the muscles to the liver and converted to glucose, which is then sent back to the muscles to provide energy. Prolonged exercise can result in significant glutamine depletion, not only because the liver uses it to produce fuel for the muscles, but also because exercise increases the demand for glutamine in the immune system cells and in tissues (particularly the gut) that use it directly.

Post-exercise glutamine depletion leaves the body more susceptible to bacterial and viral infections. Runners who maintain a proper diet and avoid overtraining are able to quickly recover normal glutamine levels, but runners who do not may develop a chronic glutamine deficit that will likely compromise performance and health. Low blood glutamine levels are commonly seen in runners suffering from overtraining syndrome, a form of chronic fatigue that affects some elite athletes.

Magnesium. Magnesium belongs to a category of minerals called electrolytes, so called because they conduct electrical signals in the body. It is found in all of the body's cells, although it is most concentrated in the bones, muscles, and soft tissues. It's a necessary element in more than 300 enzyme reactions involving nerve transmission, muscle contraction, and especially adenosine triphosphate (ATP) production. (ATP is the fundamental energy currency of the body. All other "fuels"—glucose, fats, etc.—are broken down to produce ATP, which in turn stimulates muscle contractions.)

All of the important electrolytes except calcium are lost through perspiration. Heavy sweat losses can therefore interfere with the important functions for which magnesium and other electrolytes are responsible. Low blood magnesium levels during exercise have been cited as a cause of muscle fatigue and irregular heartbeat.

Potassium. Also an electrolyte, potassium is necessary for nerve transmission, muscle contraction, and glycogen formation. It also aids in maintaining cardiovascular system function. During workouts, potassium helps calcium do its job of stimulating muscle contractions. While it is calcium that actually stimulates the contraction, it cannot do so without the aid of potassium. Excessive potassium loss through sweating can lead to heat intolerance.

Sodium/chloride. Sodium and chloride cooperate with water to help maintain the volume and balance of all the fluids outside your body's cells, such as the blood. Sodium, the best-known electrolyte, plays a particularly important role because it helps transport nutrients into cells, so they can be used for energy production as well as tissue growth and repair. In addition, sodium functions in muscle contraction and nerve impulse transmission. Excessive loss of sodium through sweating may lead to hyponatremia, a dangerous condition that I'll describe further in Chapter 5.

Vitamin E. Vitamin E serves a number of important functions in the body, but while you're running its most important job is antioxidant defense. During exercise, your body produces several times more free radicals, due to the high rate of oxygen consumption, than at rest. These free radicals attack and damage muscle cells, causing damage that impairs muscle function and leads to soreness the next day. Vitamin E is able to neutralize free radicals. Consistent training, combined with a diet rich in vitamin E, increases vitamin E storage in the body and the efficiency of its radical neutralizing actions.

Water. Water is arguably the most important nutrient of all. It accounts for two-thirds of the body's mass and is essential for a host of vital functions including proper digestion, elimination of wastes, and joint lubrication. Perhaps its most running-specific role is in perspiration, which is the body's primary cooling mechanism during running. The downside of perspiration is that the more you perspire, the more water you lose and the less efficient this cooling mechanism becomes. The loss of blood volume that comes with dehydration also hampers cardiovascular performance. Drinking water while running can limit dehydration and its effects. Drinking an enhanced water or sports drink containing electrolytes is preferable because it does a more complete job of counteracting nutrient depletion caused by perspiration.

Of these 10 nutrients discussed, 7 are able to enhance running performance when consumed during running: branched-chain and/or other amino acids, carbohydrates (from which glucose is derived), glutamine, magnesium, potassium, sodium chloride, and water. In Chapter 5, I'll give you detailed guidelines for hydration and nutrition during exercise.

USING NUTRITION TO ENHANCE POST-EXERCISE RECOVERY

Individual workouts stress your body by depleting energy supplies, disrupting muscle tissues, changing hormonal patterns, and so forth. This type of stress is often referred to as a *training stimulus*. After the workout is completed, your body initiates physiological processes designed to restore homeostasis, or the way the body was before the workout. It replenishes muscle energy stores, builds new muscle proteins, adjusts hormonal patterns, and engages in a variety of other responses. Collectively, these various processes that lead back to homeostasis are known as recovery.

There is a very close relationship between acute recovery, which is the body's short-term response to training stimuli, and adaptation, which is the body's longer-term response to repetitive training stimuli. You can think of recovery as a series of short trips that add up to the lengthy voyage of adaptation, or fitness gains.

Research has shown that nutrition after exercise has a tremendous influence on recovery. If you consume the right types and amounts of nutrients within an hour of completing a workout, your muscles will rebuild and refuel themselves much faster than if you consume the wrong nutrients or nothing at all. And because short-term recovery leads to long-term fitness adaptations, consistently practicing smart recovery nutrition will make you a better runner over time. Recovery nutrition will be our subject in Chapter 7.

USING NUTRITION TO PREVENT INJURIES AND SICKNESS

In almost every respect, runners are healthier than the population at large. There are only two small exceptions: runners experience more musculoskeletal injuries (muscle strains, bone strains, and so forth) than non-runners, and runners who train especially hard tend to suffer cold and flu more often than the average person. Nutrition can help in both of these areas.

There is evidence that proper recovery nutrition can reduce injuries by accelerating the repair of tissues damaged during running. A well-balanced overall diet that contains plenty of the various nutrients needed to make the bones, muscles, and connective tissues strong will also reduce injuries. For example, studies have shown that runners who eat too little fat experience more injuries than runners who eat more fat. Deficiencies in any of a number of other nutrients—amino acids used to rebuild damaged muscles, calcium and phosphate for bone density, and so forth—could also make you more susceptible to injury.

The best defense against cold and flu is, naturally, a strong immune system. The immune system depends on proper nutrition to function optimally. To name just a few examples of specific nutrients that support immune function, vitamin C increases antibody production; vitamin A promotes mucus production (mucus prevents foreign invaders in the body from gaining access to the bloodstream); amino acids, fats, and carbohydrate provide energy for cells of the immune system; and fatty acids produce prostaglandins, hormonelike substances some of which act as mediators in the inflammation response to infection.

Inadequate or excessive intake of certain nutrients can hamper immune defenses in various ways. In the typical American diet, the most common immunosuppressive dietary problems are excessive intake of total calories (i.e., being overweight), saturated fat, refined sugars, and caffeine.

During exercise, various aspects of immune system function are enhanced. Consistent daily exercise leads to a general strengthening of these functions. Much has been made of the fact that very intense and very long workouts temporarily suppress the immune system. However, the immunosuppressive effect of such workouts is much smaller in those who exercise regularly than in those who are sedentary. Nevertheless, while most runners experience fewer infections (cold, flu, etc.) than non-runners, there is some clinical evidence, and plenty of anecdotal evidence, that chronic heavy training slightly increases infection risk. Long-term inadequate recovery from training can lead to overtraining syndrome, a serious hormonal disorder in which depression of the immune system is often a secondary symptom.

A classic example of nutrition-exercise synergy is the fact that consuming carbohydrate during and immediately after a hard run reduces immunosuppression. David Nieman of Appalachian State University led one of several studies proving this effect. His team found that athletes who used a sports drink during exercise showed significantly reduced signs of immunosuppression afterward compared to a control group. That's one more reason to use a sports drink!

USING NUTRITION TO "IMPROVE ON NATURE"

While natural foods are the best source of nutrition for most meals and snacks, nutritional supplements are sometimes superior when it comes to meeting certain special needs that runners have. Most of the nutritional supplements marketed to athletes are useless, but a few have been proven effective in research studies. For example, creatine monohydrate is a nutritional supplement that has been shown to reduce muscle damage during long runs. Although you can get creatine from natural foods such as beef, you can't get it in amounts sufficient to match what you can get with supplementation. So this is one case where a nutritional supplement "improves on nature." I will say a lot more about creatine and a number of other nutritional supplements in Chapter 9.

CHAPTER 2

THE FOUR PRINCIPLES OF HEALTHY EATING

The average health-conscious American is a little confused about what constitutes an optimal diet. One source of that confusion is the tremendous volume of nutrition information to which we are exposed. It so permeates our culture that even those who avoid reading nutrition books and magazine articles get plenty of exposure to it. For example, just yesterday at the grocery store I grabbed a watermelon from a large crate that had a full paragraph about the merits of lycopene (a nutrient with highly touted antioxidant properties) printed on its side.

Those who conscientiously try to heed the news of each new "miracle nutrient" that's identified and every other sort of nutrition discovery that comes along can easily become overwhelmed. I imagine my fellow shoppers wandering through the supermarket aisles thinking, "Let's see, to prevent liver cancer I need carotenoids, which are in carrots; and to balance my prostaglandins I need alpha-linolenic acid, which is in salmon; and to lower my cholesterol I need plant sterols, which are in—damn it, I can't remember!" No one can retain it all, and the quantities of information we do retain are overwhelming enough to make shopping, planning meals, and eating a far more nerve-wracking set of activities than they should be.

A second source of confusion is the fact that so much of the nutrition information we get is contradictory. Why can't the nutrition authorities keep their story straight? Here are just a few of the many reasons.

Human nutrition is complex. There's just no getting around the fact that human nutrition is a breathtakingly complex subject. There are tens of thousands of biologically active chemicals at work in the human body, and almost all of them are derived from food in one way or another. Scientists are only able to study one or two small pieces of the intricate puzzle of human metabolism at a time. All too often, they are unable to observe how these pieces are affected by other, unseen pieces, and as a result they draw conclusions that will have to be retracted or revised when these other pieces come into view. Good scientists understand that all of their conclusions are tentative and subject to later revision, but we often have little choice but to base our dietary decisions on the tentative conclusions of nutrition scientists, and it can be frustrating when they are in fact changed.

One example of this dynamic is the story of margarine. In the 1960s, scientists and doctors advocated margarine as a healthier alternative to butter because margarine is lower in saturated fats than butter, and a link between saturated fat and heart disease had been recently discovered. What those doctors and scientists did not know at the time is that trans fats, of which margarine is full, are far worse. The advice to replace butter with margarine has since been retracted.

Scientists are human. While nutrition science in general can't be blamed for its piecemeal progress, individual nutrition scientists frequently commit avoidable errors that only increase our confusion once they are exposed. More often than you might think, poorly designed nutrition studies and poorly interpreted data yield false conclusions that must be corrected later. Common problems include small sample sizes, faulty data collection methods, lack of adequate placebo controls, and dismissal of unexpected results.

In some cases, studies are designed or interpreted badly with full awareness of the researchers, because they want to please the party (often a food industry corporation) funding the study. In other cases, researchers are so keen on seeing their pet hypothesis validated that, well, they *make* it right. An example of this latter scenario comes from a large, international study that sought a correlation between cholesterol levels and heart disease in 27 countries. According to the raw data there was only a weak correlation, but inexplicably, in their analysis of this data, the researchers leading the study simply threw out data from countries that defied their expectations and found a much stronger correlation in the remaining data. Years later, the correlation between total blood cholesterol levels and heart disease was proven to be much weaker than we were once led to believe.

The media exaggerates. The popular media, aware of the huge public appetite (so to speak) for nutrition information, and moving, as they do, much faster than science, frequently overhype individual studies, and thus make it seem as though the scientific understanding of the right way to eat is changing more rapidly than it actually is. Several years ago, you may recall, the media were touting soy as the ultimate superfood; a few years later, inevitably, they were hyping the dangers of eating too much soy. But if you had read only the studies on which these stories were based, you would have seen nothing like this dramatic reversal.

Anyone can give nutrition advice. A large fraction of the men and women who are given the status of nutrition experts in our society are actually nothing of the sort. Much of the dietary advice proffered by these poseurs is either repeated myth or made up completely. Bill Philips, author of the zillion-selling *Body for Life,* is a good example of a nutrition expert by reputation only. Among the pearls of wisdom dispensed in his book is the advice not to eat anything within an hour of completing a workout. I don't know where Philips got this idea, but it is one of the gravest nutrition mistakes an athlete could make, as will become abundantly clear in Chapter 7.

We have no one but ourselves to blame when we accept the likes of sitcom-actress-turned-cottage-industry magnate Suzanne Somers, putative author of *Suzanne Somers' Get Skinny on Fabulous Food,* as our nutrition oracles. But some of the fake nutrition experts are less easy to spot. For example, you might be surprised to learn that medical students typically get very little nutrition education in their four-year curriculum, yet they routinely give nutritional guidance to patients once they begin practicing. Because they did not get their knowledge of nutrition in their formal training, they get it all too often from the same place we do: the diet section of the bookstore.

Nutrition beliefs are often based on ideology. The large gaps in our scientific knowledge of human nutrition have left many an opening for ideologists of various stripes to peddle dietary philosophies based as much on politics and emotion as on fact. The immense cultural importance of food makes these philosophies very seductive to their peddlers and consumers alike. There are primitivists who contend that one should eat only raw plant foods, conspiracy theorists who view all processed foods as poisonous, food industry toadies who insist that the best foods are engineered, contrarians who are all too ready to subvert the conventional nutritional wisdom, classic conservatives who will go to any lengths to defend the majority opinion against all evidence, and other types. There will come a day when our growing scientific knowledge of human nutrition squeezes out most of the ideologists, but we're not there yet.

Sometimes greed comes before honesty. There is a lot of money to be made in selling nutrition advice and products that are based on particular kinds of nutrition advice, and sometimes there's even more money to be made when the advice is grounded in partial or complete falsehoods. The ultimate example is Robert Atkins, who almost single-handedly spawned a low-carb diet industry that peaked at $15 billion a year based on a largely bogus dietary philosophy (as we'll see in the next chapter).

It's important to understand that profit motives also color what is presented to us as nutritional fact in more insidious ways. University nutrition departments now depend heavily on large food and drug companies to fund research. (I've interviewed veteran researchers who remember when it was unthinkable to accept funding from such sources.) Even when these relationships don't affect the results of research, they affect the types of studies that are done, and are not done. Studies designed to prove that a certain product solves a health or nutrition problem are much more likely to be funded than studies that merely serve to increase our knowledge of human nutrition.

We want a magic bullet. The fake experts and profit seekers couldn't take advantage of the public so easily if not for the magic bullet–seeking mentality of the average consumer. We want to hear that there is a simple, instant, and easy dietary solution to our health and weight issues. We want the ultimate revolutionary breakthrough diet secret. Given a choice between a fake expert telling us what we want to hear and a real one giving us the same old truth, all too often we will choose to listen to the fraud. But doing so will not bring the promised results, so our sense of confusion escalates.

It is by no means wrong to want simple nutrition guidelines. In fact, nutrition guidelines have to be simple if we are to benefit from them. However, they also have to be realistic. Many of the fake experts steer us wrong by oversimplifying the actual phenomenon of human nutrition. Atkins blamed everything on carbohydrates. Peter D'Adamo reduced it all to a simple game of matching nutrition to blood type. Such diets are very simple, but their simplicity avails nothing because it derives from false ideas about nutrition. The right way to generate simple guidelines for eating is to step back from the level of specific do's and don'ts to the level of general principles. While the phenomenon of human nutrition is irreducibly complex, the core principles of healthy eating are not. By learning and focusing on the latter, you can make good nutrition choices consistently without getting bogged down in too many details.

THE FOUR PRINCIPLES OF HEALTHY EATING

In an interview, Arthur Agatston, author of the wildly successful *The South Beach Diet,* told me, "People want to be told exactly what and how much to eat every day. But it's the people who understand the principles who do well in the long term." Only when you understand the fundamental principles of healthy eating can you truly take control of your diet and avoid becoming confused by details or blown along in the direction of each new diet fad. Following are the four most fundamental principles of healthy eating. The rest is details.

PRINCIPLE #1: EAT NATURAL FOODS

Our nutritional needs are determined at the highest level by the human genome: the coded essence of our species that was fashioned through millions of years of evolution from older species. Evolution is a process by which a species continually adapts to a dynamic and changing environment, tweaking its own makeup so as to make the best use of what its environment has to offer. Food is arguably the most important component of an animal's environment. Every animal evolves in such a way as to become optimally adapted to its diet. Virtually any change in a species' food sources will necessitate further evolutionary adaptations.

Humans emerged from earlier hominid species about 1.3 million years ago. The first humans were well adapted to their diet, having evolved with it from their primate origins over a period of 2.5 million years. The diet of the first humans remains more or less the optimal human diet, because genetically we aren't much different today from our earliest ancestors. However, our modern diet differs considerably from what our ancestors ate a million years ago. This is due to the unprecedented ingenuity of our species. No other creature in the history of life on Earth has been able to manipulate its own diet to the degree we have, and in such a way as to drastically slow down our evolution by ensuring that nearly all of us survive to reach childbearing age.

The first major dietary transformation was the agricultural revolution, when we learned first how to mill and then how to cultivate cereal grains. As a result of these advances, cereal grains, which until that time had been almost completely absent in the human diet, suddenly became our primary staples. Both the variety and the amount of fruits and vegetables in the diet decreased. This happened over the course of just a few centuries—the blink of an eye on the evolutionary scale—beginning about 10,000 years ago. (The agricultural revolution and other human "advances" occurring at this time are considered so significant that they literally mark the end of an age—the Paleolithic—and the dawn of a new age—the Neolithic.) Milled whole grains are not unnatural, in any strict sense, but a grain-heavy diet is one giant step removed from the diet to which we are best adapted.

The milk of domesticated animals also entered the human diet at this time. Milk and other dairy products are nutritionally very different from most other foods because of their high levels of saturated fat and extreme caloric density. Genetically, we are not well adapted to eating dairy foods, and indeed a quarter of human adults cannot even digest milk properly. While the other three-quarters of us can digest milk, the main problem with eating a lot of dairy foods is that it boosts our total intake of saturated fat and overall calories unnaturally, leading to overweight and "diseases of affluence" such as diabetes and heart disease.

The second major transformation in the human diet began with the industrial revolution and continues today. The speed and thoroughness with which our food has changed within just the past 150 years makes the agricultural revolution look like nothing at all. As a result, the so-called modern Western diet is highly unnatural in a number of important ways. Today, grains and grain-based foods remain staples in our diets, but most of them are highly processed. Pesticides, many of them toxic to humans, are used on most of the plant foods we eat. Livestock raised for meat are genetically modified (as are a growing number of plant foods), pumped full of growth hormones and antibiotics, and fed highly unnatural diets of their own; much of our farmed fish is produced in a similar way. Oils are extracted from plants and refined with bleaches, detergents, and solvents. These oils are then added to many of our processed foods and used for frying, which further damages the oils. Natural and artificial preservatives are also added to many processed foods. The list goes on.

Thousands upon thousands of scientific studies have shown that this unnatural diet comes with many severe health consequences. And anything that's bad for your health is bad for your running. If your health and running are important to you, I strongly encourage you to make your diet more natural than the average American diet in certain key ways.

Eat more fresh fruits and vegetables. If you had a nickel for every time someone advised you to eat more fruits and vegetables, you could pay off the US federal deficit (supposing you were so inclined). There are good reasons to keep up this drumbeat. Fresh fruits and vegetables were the main foods in the diet of our oldest ancestors, and their hominid ancestors, and their primate ancestors. Consequently, our optimal health today depends on our eating at least eight servings of fruits and vegetables daily. In addition to providing carbohydrates for energy, fiber for digestion and elimination, and vitamins and minerals for a long list of functions, fruits and vegetables give us a vast variety of so-called phytonutrients that are now understood to constitute a critical part of our antioxidant defenses. Animal foods do not contain phytonutrients, and whole grains contain them in much smaller amounts than fruits and vegetables.

Phytonutrients are a terrific example of how thoroughly adapted the human genome is to our ancestral diet. Unlike the essential vitamins and minerals, phytonutrients are not strictly necessary for our survival. They are not indispensable ingredients of any cell or irreplaceable substrates of any critical metabolic process. However, many phytonutrients are powerful antioxidants able to prevent and limit damage to DNA, cell membranes, and tissues caused by free radicals, toxins, and foreign invaders. (Some phytonutrients do not act as antioxidants but assist us in other ways, for example by activating key enzymes.) Scientists now believe that fruits and vegetables have a preventive effect against 16 types of cancer. Because free radical damage plays a major role in aging, phytonutrients almost surely slow general bodily deterioration and increase the lifespan.

For runners, phytonutrients also promote faster post-workout recovery and tissue healing and reduce the risk of injuries, sickness, and overtraining, as antioxidants play a role in each of these areas.

Eat fewer processed grains. It was bad enough for human health when grains largely replaced fruits and vegetables (and in some places, meat) in the diet of our Neolithic ancestors in approximately 8,000

GET YOUR PHYTONUTRIENTS HERE!

A couple of years ago, scientists representing the US Department of Agriculture picked the top 20 best sources of antioxidants. Here's their list. I wouldn't take the specific order too seriously—the ranking was mainly a marketing gimmick—but what's certain is that most or all of these foods should have a place in your diet.

1. Small red beans (dried)
2. Wild blueberries
3. Red kidney beans
4. Pinto beans
5. Blueberries (cultivated)
6. Cranberries
7. Artichokes (cooked)
8. Blackberries
9. Prunes
10. Raspberries
11. Strawberries
12. Red Delicious apples
13. Granny Smith apples
14. Pecans
15. Sweet cherries
16. Black plums
17. Russet potatoes (cooked)
18. Black beans (dried)
19. Plums
20. Gala apples

BC. Grains are a lot less nutrient-dense than most fruits and vegetables, so they provide narrower support for our overall health. At the same time, grains tend to be substantially more energy-dense (i.e., calorically dense) than fruits and vegetables, so they are more likely to contribute to weight gain, especially when combined with low activity levels. But our big switch from eating mostly whole grains to eating mostly refined grains within the past 150 years has been infinitely worse for our health. Foods made with processed grains tend to be even less nutrient-dense and more calorie-dense. The worst foods are the ones that are full of refined sugar (e.g., sucrose, corn syrup) and those that contain both refined flour and processed oils (e.g., hydrogenated or partially hydrogenated vegetable oil).

It's unrealistic to ask most people to eliminate these foods from their diet, but you must try to limit them. There are lots of simple ways to replace refined grain foods with whole grain alternatives. If you eat breakfast cereal, switch from Froot Loops to Wheaties or some other whole grain cereal. If you eat bread, switch from white bread to whole wheat bread. If your diet relies heavily on grains in general, replace some of them with fruits and vegetables. (Replace refined grains first, whole grains second.) Instead of having a side of french bread with your dinner, have a side of baked beans. Instead of cereal for breakfast, have a grilled vegetable omelet.

Eat fewer processed and damaged oils. Of the three basic types of fats (saturated, monounsaturated, and polyunsaturated), which I'll discuss in greater depth in the next chapter, polyunsaturated fats are by far the least stable. Industrial processing, heating, and even plain old oxygen can damage these oils, transforming them from healthful nutrients into toxic "anti-nutrients" (i.e., nutrients that do more harm than good in the body in any amount). Prior to the nineteenth century, most of the polyunsaturated fats in the diet were consumed in their natural form. This is no longer the case.

Major sources of damaged oils are fried foods, processed snacks and baked goods, butter substitutes, roasted nuts, and cooking oils other than olive oil. These foods should have a very small place in your diet. Good sources of undamaged polyunsaturated oils include olive oil, fresh nuts and seeds, wild salmon, and soy.

Eat more organic foods. Organic foods are plant and animal foods produced in somewhat old-fashioned ways that forsake some of the modern technological shortcuts that make foods less healthy. Organic fruits and vegetables are produced without the use of chemical agents (pesticides, fungicides, etc.) and usually in much naturally richer soil than nonorganic plant foods (that is, soil with more minerals and only natural fertilizers). These chemical agents, all used to kill things that kill plants, are toxic by definition. For example, methyl bromide, a commonly used fungicide, is also a known carcinogen. Chemical residues remain on the surface of fruits and vegetables until you eat them, unless you peel and/or thoroughly wash them. The agricultural industry insists that the small amounts of pesticide residues on their foods are not enough to cause health problems, but they would say so whether it was true or not, and we really don't know that it's not.

No food can be more nutritious than its own food source is, and numerous studies have shown that the nutrient-poor soil in which most nonorganic plants are grown yields fruits and vegetables with lesser amounts of vitamins, minerals, and phytonutrients. In addition to being healthier, organic fruits and vegetables also usually taste better. The downside is that they are more expensive and less accessible and they often spoil faster. But your health is worth a little money and inconvenience, so choose organic fruits and vegetables over nonorganic ones whenever possible.

Organic meats (and eggs and dairy products) come from animals that are raised on organic grains or grasses, are able to move about freely during their lifetime, and have not been injected with antibiotics or growth hormones. There is a great deal of debate about whether the use of antibiotics and hormones makes animal foods more or less dangerous to the health of those who eat them. Without even getting into that debate, I'd just like to point out that the previously-mentioned rule about the food your food eats applies here, too. Organic meats, eggs, and dairy products tend to be more nutritious because the diet of the animals they come from is also more nutritious. This is especially true of grass-fed animals, whose products typically contain much higher levels of omega-3 fatty acids (whose benefits are described in the next chapter) and much less saturated fat.

I recommend that you buy organic versions of all food types whenever possible. This goes for boxed and canned foods and other packaged foods as well. In addition to containing organically produced ingredients, such products do not contain most of the unhealthy additives (artificial colorings, preservatives, etc.) that are common in their nonorganic counterparts. Among the most important additives to avoid are the following:

- Artificial colors (especially red dye No. 40, blue dye No. 1, and yellow dye No. 5)
- Artificial sweeteners (especially aspartame)
- Preservatives including nitrites, nitrates, sulfites, MSG (monosodium glutamate), aluminum, BHA, BHT, and TBHQ
- Hydrogenated and brominated oils

All of these ingredients are associated with health risks. Avoid them whenever possible in nonorganic foods, too. As a more general rule, when buying packaged foods, choose those with the fewest and most familiar ingredients. The ingredients list of any packaged product you buy regularly should look similar to the recipe you would use to make the same thing at home.

WHAT'S A SERVING?

Here are some examples of what counts as a complete serving of various foods.

Apple	1 small apple
Banana	½ medium banana
Broccoli	1 cup raw, ½ cup cooked
Green beans	1 cup raw, ½ cup cooked
Grapefruit	½ medium grapefruit
Orange	1 small orange
Peach	1 small peach
Spinach	1 cup raw, ½ cup cooked
Strawberries	1¼ cups
Tomato	½ medium tomato (4–6 slices)
All meats	2–3 ounces cooked
Bread	1 slice
Fish	2–3 ounces cooked
Milk	1 cup
Pasta	½ cup cooked
Yogurt	1 cup

PRINCIPLE #2: EAT A BALANCE AND A VARIETY OF FOODS

Perhaps the most characteristic feature of the human diet as compared to the diets of other species is the sheer variety of foods we eat. When our ancestors diverged from chimpanzees more than four million years ago, the key trend in the evolution of our diet, which paralleled our genetic evolution, was a trend toward incorporating more and more foods. Paleolithic humans (living between 10,000 and 8,000 BC) are believed to have consumed anywhere from 100 to 200 different plant foods annually.

The agricultural revolution and other historical events sharply reduced the variety in the human diet, but the more recent trend of global trade has introduced a new opportunity for dietary variety. We now have unprecedented access to plant and animal foods indigenous to every part of the globe. It's a good idea to take full advantage of this access to maintain a highly varied diet. This will go a long way toward ensuring that you get neither too much nor too little of any particular nutrient.

There are two levels of dietary balance. The first level is types of food. There are various ways to categorize food types, but the following list is as good as any: vegetables, fruits, grains, legumes (beans), nuts and seeds, meat and eggs, poultry, seafood, and dairy foods. Ideally, your diet will include all of these foods. Maintaining an optimum balance among these food types does not mean you should eat all of them in equal amounts. Vegetables (including legumes) and fruits should have the largest place at eight to 10 servings a day. Whether you eat more (whole) grains than nondairy animal foods or vice versa is not important and therefore a matter of personal choice, but a fairly even balance between these categories is a good place to start. Consumption of dairy foods generally should not exceed three servings a day.

It's also a good idea to eat for variety within each food category, and especially within the vegetable and fruit categories. Different fruits and vegetables often have very different phytonutrient profiles, so the fewer types you eat, the more phytonutrients you miss out on. Color is a good guide, because phytonutrients give plant foods their distinctive colors. The more colorful your diet is, the better. Variation within the other food categories is not quite as important but still highly beneficial to the goal of achieving optimal nutrient balance. So, the meat you eat should not always be chicken; your grain should not always be wheat.

BALANCING FOOD TYPES

There is no perfect formula that can tell you precisely how many servings from each food category you should eat daily, but you can't go wrong by following these general guidelines, which are informed by both nutrition science and our cultural preferences.

Food Category	Recommended Servings per Day
Vegetables	4–5
Fruits	3–5
Whole grains	6–8
Legumes, beans, nuts and seeds	4–5
Dairy	3
Lean meats, poultry, eggs	1–2
Fish	3–6 (per week)

It takes a little work to maintain a well-varied diet. However, the great thing about focusing on consuming a variety and balance of natural food types is that it allows you to achieve a highly nutritious diet without even thinking about nutrients—indeed, without even having to know the first thing about the nutrients that any given food contains. Just like our Paleolithic ancestors.

PRINCIPLE #3: BALANCE YOUR ENERGY INTAKE WITH YOUR ENERGY NEEDS

Beyond all of the changes in the content of our diet, there has also been a tremendous change since the Neolithic Age in the amount of energy we spend attaining food. As hunter-gatherers, we had to do a great deal of physical work to produce and acquire food. With the onset of the agricultural revolution, the labor requirement decreased markedly, and in the industrial age it has plummeted. In the twenty-first century only a few of us produce our own food, and acquiring it entails nothing more than a drive to the supermarket. In fact, if we want to, we can "work" in front of a computer all day at home and have all of our food delivered straight to the front door. I don't know anyone personally who actually goes quite so far, but apparently it is a growing trend in metropolitan areas, and the lifestyle of the average white-collar worker comes alarmingly close to this extreme.

Our hunter-gatherer ancestors often had a hard time getting enough calories to supply their energy needs. Our own problem is the opposite. As runners we are better off than most people, but even for many of us, maintaining a lean body composition is challenging.

Conceptually, it's very simple. If you're currently at or very near your optimal body composition, your goal is to consume the same number of calories in food as you release through metabolism and activity each day. If you are currently carrying too much fat on your body, your goal is to consume slightly (100 to 500) fewer calories in food than you release through metabolism and activity each day until you reach your optimum body composition. You can lose weight faster by drastically cutting calories, but the hunger will drive you mad and the resulting energy deficit will ruin your workouts and severely compromise your recovery. A slightly negative caloric balance is more manageable and healthier.

One way to find the right balance is to estimate how many calories you consume in food and how many you burn daily and then adjust your diet accordingly. (I don't usually advise performance-minded runners to adjust their training for the sake of creating a caloric deficit.) Dietitians and weight loss counselors often help their clients do this, but the only convenient means of generating these estimates are actually quite inaccurate. Nevertheless, going through the process is an excellent way to become more aware of what (and how much) you're eating, which in itself is proven to facilitate fat loss.

A simpler way to create a slight caloric deficit is to take your current eating habits as a starting point and make a handful of targeted changes designed to trim calories and make better use of the calories you do consume. To ensure that these targeted changes are adequate, regularly monitor your body composition. As I discuss in Chapter 4, body composition is an excellent indicator of health and fitness, whereas body weight is a rather poor one.

In addition to balancing your energy intake with your energy needs from day to day, it is also beneficial to balance your energy intake with your energy needs over the course of any given day. Doing so ensures that you have the energy you need to perform well in your daily tasks, including workouts, throughout the day. In this regard, eating smaller meals more frequently is better than eating fewer, larger meals. Eating some kind of breakfast is especially important. Include a source of carbohydrate in each meal and snack. If you include high glycemic index carbohydrates (i.e., quickly digested carbohydrates) in your snacks or meals (see examples in the next chapter), be sure to include some fat and/or protein as well, as this will slow absorption of the carbs so that the energy they provide lasts longer. Exceptions are pre-workout and post-workout meals and snacks, when high GI carbs are preferable.

PRINCIPLE #4: CUSTOMIZE YOUR DIET TO YOUR INDIVIDUAL NEEDS

Until this point, I've been writing as though our prehistoric ancestors in all parts of the globe ate the same way. The evidence clearly shows they did not. While I can assure you that none of them ate french fries or drank soft drinks, there were significant differences in the natural foods available geographically in various human environments. This undoubtedly led to some race-specific genetic adaptations that entail race-specific nutritional needs and requirements.

While we know a fair amount about how diets differed in various parts of the world in prehistory, we don't yet know much about how actual nutritional needs may differ based on racial origin. It's not unlikely that these differences are much smaller than the differences in ancestral diets, because the human species in general has a great ability to adapt to different types of diet. Some diet gurus have tried to make a quick buck by pretending they know much more about race-based differences in nutritional needs than anyone really does, and by exaggerating these differences. Don't listen to them!

More important than race-based differences in nutritional needs are simple genetic variations (called polymorphisms) that exist in individuals of every race and that affect nutritional needs. Individual genetic variation can influence how nutrients are assimilated, metabolized, stored, and excreted by the body. This means the perfect diet for you might not be the perfect diet for me.

Food allergies and intolerances are an obvious example of how genetic variations can affect nutritional needs. A food allergy occurs when the immune system mistakenly views a certain nutrient as a threat to the body. A food intolerance occurs when nutrients in a particular food cause some other kind of abnormal negative reaction in the body. More than 25 percent of the world's adults are lactose intolerant, meaning their bodies lose the ability to synthesize the enzyme needed to metabolize lactose (milk sugar) after infancy. The most common food allergies are to milk (this is unrelated to lactose intolerance), eggs, peanuts, tree nuts (walnuts, cashews, etc.), fish, shellfish, soy, and wheat.

Beyond allergies and intolerances, there are many other kinds of differences in nutritional needs, not all of them well understood. One diet-related genetic variation that has received a lot of attention lately is a predisposition for metabolic syndrome, a cluster of metabolic abnormalities that include insulin resistance, glucose intolerance, high

(continued on page 40)

SAMPLE FOOD JOURNAL FORMAT

Keeping a food journal is a great way to figure out how your diet is affecting your health and your running. It usually takes a minimum of 3 days to identify a pattern. If you make a change to your eating habits based on a pattern you observe, continue journaling for at least 3 more days to determine the effects of the change.

Meals When? What? How much?	2 Hours Later Appetite? Energy? Mental clarity? Mood?
Meal 1 6:30 am ½ cup old-fashioned oatmeal with dried cranberries and 1 tablespoon honey 8 ounces orange juice 12 ounces coffee	Not hungry; energy level and concentration good; mood a little low.
Meal 2	
Meal 3	
Meal 4	
Meal 5	
Meal 6 (or last meal of the day)	Slept well for 8 hours.

If you eat fewer than six meals in a day, leave the irrelevant boxes blank and record your sleep quality in the box to the right of your last meal of the day. Likewise, leave all of the boxes blank in the "Subsequent Workout" column except the one that shares a row with the meal that preceded your daily workout.

	Subsequent Workout Energy? GI troubles? Focus? Attitude?
	Easy 40-minute run; felt very strong; finished feeling refreshed.

blood pressure, high blood triglycerides, and high levels of abdominal fat. Metabolic syndrome is generally considered a lifestyle condition because it can easily be prevented through proper diet and exercise, but genetic predisposition is nevertheless the primary cause—bad lifestyle habits are the trigger.

"Nutrigenomics" is a name that's recently been given to the medical practice of customizing diet to the genetic needs of the individual. While it holds much promise for the future, it is as yet a very primitive form of medicine, despite what you may be led to believe by a growing number of companies that offer genetic nutritional profiles based on analysis of a personal DNA sample (usually a cheek swab) that you submit to them. These are scams.

The best way to customize your diet to your individual needs (in the absence of major nutrition-related health problems) is by keeping a food journal. First, modify your diet according to the first three rules described in this chapter. It's OK and perhaps best to do this gradually, step by step, especially if your current eating habits leave much to be desired. Once you're eating more or less by the rules, start keeping a food journal that includes everything you eat and drink and how your body responds to it. Note how you feel 2 hours after the meal, how you perform in your next workout, and how you sleep at night after your last meal of the day. A few examples of possible problems you might observe are postmeal sluggishness, general fatigue, poor workout performance, gastrointestinal problems during workouts, constipation, headaches, insomnia, mood swings, and heartburn. (See the example of a food journal in the sidebar on pages 38 to 39.)

Once you've isolated a problem, modify your diet in a sensible way and see if it resolves the issue. For example, if you experience afternoon headaches, it's possible that you're failing to rehydrate properly after workouts. Increase your post-workout fluid intake and see what happens. Sometimes your first hunch will pay off. Other times you'll have to do a little research into the potential dietary causes of the issue you're having and perhaps try a few changes before you find the true fix. (It's beyond the scope of this book to discuss all the possibilities, as there are hundreds.) In still other cases you'll need to seek the help of a dietitian or physician.

Ultimately, most of the responsibility for finding your own optimal eating patterns falls to you. The universal guidelines for healthy eating described in this chapter will get you most of the way there. However, some nutritional needs are not universal but are particular to those who share certain genetic polymorphisms. This reality is seen in virtually every clinical nutritional experiment performed. While it's almost always the average result that's reported, responses are invariably quite disparate throughout the pool of subjects. Therefore, it's important that you treat your own diet as a continually unfolding experiment. Always pay close attention to what you eat and drink and how it seems to affect you. Don't be afraid to try various changes when something isn't working. In this way you might never find the perfect diet, but you will move ever closer to it.

CHAPTER 3

BALANCING YOUR ENERGY SOURCES

I am not a practicing sports nutritionist, but I consult one. Her name is Kim Mueller-Brown. When Kim first analyzed my diet, I was shocked to discover that I did not balance my energy sources—carbohydrates, fats, and proteins— the way I thought I did. I had considered myself an abject carb-guzzler, aiming to get 60 percent of my daily calories from carbohydrate, the general recommendation for endurance athletes. As it turned out, only 50 percent of my calories came from carbs.

I was also dismayed because I assumed that this "deficit" must be bad for my running. But on further reflection, I realized that I could not identify a single negative consequence of this "deficit." My workout performances were right on target, and I was recovering well from training. So I still maintain a diet that's 50 percent carbohydrate, and I'm still running well. As they say, "If it ain't broke, don't fix it."

The lesson I learned from this experience is that runners need not rely on strict formulas to balance our energy sources. Consequently, I no longer use formulas in advising other runners how to balance their carbs, fats, and proteins. Instead, I encourage them to find the balance that works best for them.

This is not to suggest that anything goes. To achieve optimal performance nutrition, it is essential that you balance your energy sources properly. What does this mean? First of all, you need to consume the right amount of carbohydrate, fat, and protein—neither too much nor too little. You must also consume these nutrients in the right proportions relative to one another. When you give one of them too large a place in your diet, at least one of the other two will be crowded out, which is always problematic, regardless of whether it's carbohydrate, fat, or protein that is neglected. Finally, there are various types and sources of carbohydrates, fats, and proteins, and you need to balance these as well.

This may sound difficult, but it's not. The idea is simply to consume the nutrients in a way that corresponds with the six pillars of performance nutrition described in Chapter 1 and the four principles of healthy eating described in Chapter 2. To review, the six pillars suggest that you use nutrition to enhance your general health, maximize your body's adaptations to training, fuel running performance, enhance post-exercise recovery, prevent injuries and sickness, and "improve on nature." The four principles of healthy eating are to eat natural foods, eat a balance and variety of foods, match your energy intake with your energy needs, and customize your diet to meet your individual needs. Let's take a closer look at what carbohydrates, fats, and proteins are and what they do.

MEET YOUR ENERGY SOURCES

As I'm sure you know, three types of nutrients serve as energy sources in the body: carbohydrates, fats, and proteins. Together these energy sources are classified as macronutrients ("macro" is Greek for large) because we need them in very large amounts compared to vitamins, minerals, and other nutrients. (Water, which provides no energy, is the only nutrient we need in greater quantity.) The body uses carbohydrates almost exclusively for energy. Fats are used primarily for energy, but also in other important ways. Proteins are used primarily for functions other than energy provision, yet they still provide about 15 percent of the body's energy at rest.

Nutrient energy and metabolic energy (i.e., body energy) are most often measured in calories. Thus, to say we get all of our energy from carbohydrates, fats, and proteins is to say we get all of our calories from these three nutrients.

CARBOHYDRATES: PURE ENERGY

As their name suggests, carbohydrates are compounds made up of carbon and hydrogen, plus oxygen, which are arranged into ring-shaped molecules called monosaccharides (single sugars). These rings link together to form larger and more complex carbohydrates. The largest carbohydrates contain many thousands of linked sugars. They are abundant in most plant foods, especially fruits and grains. Only one carbohydrate, lactose (the sugar in milk), is actually made by the body.

While the variety of individual carbohydrate types is great, nearly all of them are broken down into glucose (the simplest of all sugars) in the stomach, intestine, and liver. Glucose is the only form of carbohydrate (besides glycogen, which is simply stored chains of glucose) that tissues of the body can metabolize to produce ATP—the body's fundamental energy currency. Glucose is transported through the blood to the tissues and organs that use it as a fuel. The major glucose users are the brain, the liver, the skeletal muscles, the kidneys, and red blood cells. If glucose entering the blood from the liver is not needed for immediate energy, much of it is stored in the muscles and liver as glycogen (short-term storage) or converted to fats (specifically, triglycerides) and deposited in adipose tissue (long-term storage). Some types of cells, including skeletal muscle cells, require insulin to absorb glucose. Other cell types, such as brain cells, are able to draw glucose straight from the blood.

The liver and the pancreas cooperate to maintain blood glucose levels within the narrow healthy range required for the body's optimal function. When the blood glucose level rises, as it does after a high-carbohydrate meal, the pancreas reacts by releasing insulin, which delivers glucose to the tissues that need it, thereby returning the blood glucose level to the center of the normal range. When the body loses its ability to properly clear excess glucose from the blood, as in diabetes, there are serious health consequences including damage to the arteries that may ultimately lead to heart disease.

The blood glucose level only falls below the healthy range—a condition called hypoglycemia—in extreme circumstances such as starvation and exhaustive exercise. The liver stores enough glycogen to keep the blood glucose level normal for a full 24 hours even without carbohydrate intake. In addition, the liver can synthesize glucose from amino acids and lipids (i.e., fats), which are always available in an almost unlimited supply.

Many people believe that blood glucose levels fluctuate wildly throughout the day, skyrocketing after high-carbohydrate meals and plummeting between meals, but in healthy individuals they actually don't. Nevertheless, the brain is so keenly sensitive to small fluctuations in blood glucose that we experience undeniable "sugar rushes" (bursts of energy) shortly after eating sugary snacks and "blood sugar crashes" (fatigue, poor concentration, and lethargy) an hour or two later, even though the actual fluctuations in blood glucose levels are small.

Unlike fats, carbohydrates cannot be stored in large amounts; unlike proteins, they are not used structurally (i.e., they don't serve as material components of cells). Instead, they are continually burned, so the body needs a steady supply of them from the diet. A sedentary individual needs to consume about 3 grams of carbohydrate per pound of body weight daily to replace what his or her body burns. Athletes and people who exercise regularly need to consume up to 5 grams per pound to meet daily energy needs. (There are slightly more than 4 calories of energy in 1 gram of carbohydrate.)

A diet that does not contain enough carbohydrate is likely to have several functional and health consequences. One of them is muscle wasting. This occurs when muscle proteins are broken down to provide amino acids, which can be converted into glucose to make up for the lack of glucose provided by dietary carbohydrate. Except in cases of malnutrition and starvation, very low carbohydrate intake is usually made up for with very high fat and/or protein intake, which leads to other sorts of problems. Eating too much fat, for example, can weaken the immune system. Excessive carbohydrate consumption is equally problematic. It can lead to high levels of fat storage, insulin insensitivity, and glycation (abnormal reactions between glucose and tissue proteins that contribute to atherosclerosis and accelerated aging).

Different varieties of carbohydrate are digested differently. Most but not all simple sugars are digested quickly and easily, resulting in a rapid influx of glucose into the bloodstream. This is beneficial when you need quick energy, but not when you need sustained energy. One example of a simple sugar that is more resistant to digestion than others is fructose, the main sugar in fruit.

Starches, a more complex carbohydrate, are more or less the plant equivalent of glycogen in the sense that they store glucose for later use. The major difference is that many vegetables can store very large amounts of starch. The digestibility of any given vegetable depends largely on whether it contains mostly amylase starch (which is harder to digest) or amylopectin starch (which is easier to digest). Some foods that contain significant amounts of starch include potatoes, wheat, rice, and other grains. White rice contains a lot of amylopectin and is easier to digest and consequently provides quicker energy; brown rice contains a lot of amylase, is digested more slowly, and provides longer lasting energy.

Fiber (also known as roughage) is the name given to two kinds of highly complex carbohydrate that are totally indigestible. Insoluble fiber (mainly cellulose) serves as an important structural material in plants. It does not provide nutrition to humans but benefits us instead by absorbing and neutralizing toxins and by contributing to well-hydrated, bulky solid waste that is easily passed. Water-soluble fiber helps the body absorb minerals and helps remove nutrient excesses, including cholesterol, from the body. Examples of fiber-rich foods are whole grains, green leafy vegetables, and beans.

Although fiber is a carbohydrate, it provides no calories (energy) because it is not absorbed into the bloodstream. In this book, when I refer to carbohydrate, I am generally referring specifically to the sugars and starches that do provide calories.

FATS: A LITTLE GOES A LONG WAY

The term "fat" is often used as a synonym for lipids, but technically speaking, fats are one class of lipids, which also include oils and more complex compounds such as cholesterol. All fats and oils are composed of fatty acids, which are usually linked in three-unit molecules called triglycerides. Ninety-five percent of the fats consumed in the diet are triglycerides.

There are three major types of fatty acids: saturated, monounsaturated, and polyunsaturated. They are distinguished from one another by the nature of their molecular bonds and the number of hydrogen atoms they contain. (Like carbohydrates, fatty acids are made up of carbon, hydrogen, and oxygen.) Saturated fats are very stable, typically solid at room temperature, and are found in the greatest abundance in meats and dairy foods. Monounsaturated fats are liquid at room temperature and are most concentrated in oils such as olive oil, peanut oil, and canola oil. Polyunsaturated fats are unstable and are also most abundant in certain plant oils—particularly corn and soybean oils—as well as in seeds, whole grains, and fatty types of fish (e.g., salmon and tuna). Because of their instability, polyunsaturated fats oxidize (i.e., turn rancid) very easily. Polyunsaturated oils are oxidized by frying, heating, and exposure to light and air. Oxidized oils cause free radical damage to body tissues, so it's important to get your polyunsaturated fats as much as possible from nonoxidized sources.

Trans fatty acids (aka trans fats) are a form of polyunsaturated-turned-saturated fat that are not healthy in any amount. They are essentially man-made fats produced through food industry processing (although they do occur naturally in very small quantities). The heating and bleaching processes by which oils such as corn and safflower are extracted from seeds create many trans fats. Trans fats are also a product of hydrogenation, a chemical process by which hydrogen is added to polyunsaturated fatty acids to create a solid, spreadable fat with increased shelf life. They are found in many packaged, processed baked goods and snack foods. Research has shown that trans fats harden arteries, increase "bad" cholesterol and lower "good" cholesterol, and increase the risk of heart attack, stroke, and brain aneurysm. They may also contribute to other degenerative diseases including some cancers. In a word, trans fats are essentially poisonous.

Some polyunsaturated fats are also known as essential fatty acids because our bodies need them but cannot make them from other nutrients. The essential fatty acids are, specifically, linoleic acid, which belongs to the omega-3 series, and linolenic acid, which belongs to the omega-6 series. Omega-6 fatty acids are abundant in many seed and nut oils and in animal fat. (Although no animal can synthesize linoleic acid, animals that eat plant foods containing it wind up storing it in their fat tissue.) Omega-3 fatty acids are harder to come by naturally in this day and age. They're found in high amounts in nonfarmed salmon, organic (grass-fed) meats and eggs, walnuts, sardines, and flax seeds. Dark, leafy greens, soybeans, and some other foods have them in modest amounts. Most Americans do not eat enough omega-3 fats.

Fats serve a whole host of functions in the body. They are the most energy-dense macronutrient (at 9 calories per gram) and they provide many of the body's tissues and organs (including the heart) with most of their energy. All cell membranes are made up of a type of fat known as phospholipids. Fats are also components of some hormones and of chemicals that control blood clotting and muscle contractions, and they provide insulation and protection for nerves. Saturated and monounsaturated fats are used mainly for energy, while polyunsaturated fats are used mainly in cell membranes and hormones.

When fat contributes fewer than 15 percent of calories in the diet, the body usually does not function optimally. Problems can include immunosuppression, low energy, and depressed moods. Running performance will also suffer. Inadequate fat consumption lowers the production and activity of fat-burning enzymes, decreasing fat-burning efficiency during running and thereby lessening endurance. Studies have also shown that runners who consume the least fat have a higher risk of injury than runners who eat moderate or relatively high amounts of fat. This is probably because runners who eat too little fat do not get enough nutrition to adequately repair the microscopic muscle damage that occurs during running.

While dietary fat deficiency is rare, deficiency in omega-3 fats, as mentioned, is widespread. Research has shown that a good balance of omega-6 and omega-3 fats is needed for balance in the production of prostaglandins—hormones that play key roles in everything from cell growth and differentiation to immune function. One of many possible consequences of omega-6/omega-3 imbalance in runners is compromised recovery. Omega-6 fats help generate prostaglandins that promote inflammation, while omega-3 fats generate anti-inflammatory prostaglandins. Inflammation in muscle tissue following exercise is a cause of what is called secondary muscle damage, which is the main reason you wake up sore the morning after an especially hard run. Therefore, a diet that's too low in omega-3 fats may slow muscle repair between workouts.

Since carbohydrate usually fills the caloric gap, very low-fat diets can also lead to the above-mentioned functional and health problems associated with excessive carbohydrate consumption. Excessive fat consumption, like excessive carbohydrate consumption, often causes high levels of fat storage and all the functional and health problems that come with it.

PROTEINS: WHAT WE'RE MADE OF

The building blocks of human proteins are 20 amino acids that are obtained from both plant and animal sources. Their main ingredient is nitrogen, which is not present in carbohydrates and lipids. The amino acids are strung together in various combinations to create tens of thousands of distinct proteins, each with its own set of functions in the body. Protein synthesis is governed at its highest level by our DNA.

Of the 20 amino acids, 9 are considered to be essential, meaning the body cannot make them, so they must be obtained from the diet. The remaining, nonessential amino acids can be synthesized using carbohydrates and fats. The human body does not use any intact dietary proteins consumed in foods. Instead, it always breaks them down into their constituent amino acids (or groups of amino acids called peptides) and then makes new proteins wherever they are needed in the body.

Protein is the basic structural material of all organ and tissue cells. There are also many biologically active proteins in the body, including enzymes, antibodies, hormones, neurotransmitters, nutrient transport and storage compounds, and cell membrane receptors. In addition, amino acids released from proteins can serve as direct and indirect energy sources, although this is not their preferred use except in a few cases (e.g., glutamine in the gut).

There is no storage site for amino acids in the body. Ninety-nine percent of the amino acids inside us at any given time are contained in proteins. However, proteins are in a state of continual turnover. A typical protein exists for no more than several hours before it is broken down and its amino acids are used to create one or more new proteins. This high rate of turnover allows the body to adjust quickly to changes in the internal environment, remodel tissue for growth and repair, and destroy faulty proteins before they cause major problems.

Because amino acids are highly recyclable, our dietary protein requirements are rather small, despite the fact that protein accounts for about 20 percent of a typical person's body mass (75 percent of non-water mass). A nonathletic adult requires about half a gram of protein per pound of body weight per day to replace the small amount of essential amino acids that are metabolized irreversibly. Runners lose more essential amino acids as a result of training, so their protein needs are a little higher: up to 0.9 gram per pound per day.

Animal foods contain the highest amounts of protein. They also contain the proteins that are most like our own, so they are more "bioavailable"—that is, more easily used inside the body. Nevertheless, there are plenty of protein-rich plant foods. These include nuts, seeds, and some beans (especially soybeans). Vegetarians—and particularly vegetarian athletes—need to work a little harder to get enough protein, but it's not impossible. There are many highly accomplished vegetarian runners. In fact, meat has a very small place in

HOW MUCH CARBOHYDRATE, FAT, AND PROTEIN DOES A RUNNER NEED?

These ranges are a little broader than those given by most sports nutrition experts. The reason is simply that a wide range of macronutrient breakdowns has been shown to be equally effective in athletes. Most runners have some ability to adapt to various balances, but many feel and perform best on a diet skewed toward one extreme or the other of these ranges. You may need to experiment to find the balance that's best for you.

	As a Percentage of Total Calories	Adjusted for Body Weight
Carbohydrate	40–70%	3–5 g/lb
Fat	20–40%	0.7–1.4 g/lb
Protein	15–25%	0.6–0.9 g/lb

the Kenyan and Ethiopian diets, which fuel a hugely disproportionate number of the world's best runners.

Americans are much more likely to eat too much protein than too little. The average American gets twice the recommended protein intake on a daily basis, largely because of our heavy reliance on animal foods. The human body cannot absorb more than about 1 gram of protein per pound of body weight daily. Eating more than this amount of protein crowds out the other macronutrients and also causes dehydration and leeches minerals such as calcium from the bones.

While protein undernutrition is rare among runners, it is not unheard of. The consequences of even a mild deficiency may include poor recovery, susceptibility to infections, and frequent injuries. More common than protein deficiency in runners in heavy training is deficiency in the amino acid glutamine, which is used at high rates during exercise.

BALANCING THE MACRONUTRIENTS

The primary source of information about macronutrients in our society is, unfortunately, diet books. Even lean runners and others who don't read such books get much of their information about macronutrients from diet books indirectly through those who do. Each of the successful diet books has a defining shtick, and invariably the shtick is grounded in some sort of macronutrient formula. These formulas are all over the map. *The Zone Diet* advocates a breakdown of 40 percent carbohydrate, 30 percent fat, and 30 percent protein. *Dr. Atkins' New Diet Revolution* prescribes a low-carbohydrate diet. *The Perricone Prescription* recommends a low-fat diet.

Is there truly a perfect macronutrient formula? If so, which is it? As you'll see in the following sections on how much carbohydrate, fat, and protein you need, most humans are able to function well on a variety of macronutrient ratios. For most of us, there is a broad acceptable range of carbohydrate, fat, and protein consumption. What's more important is that you get each of these nutrients from good sources.

Some people are less able to adapt to different macronutrient balances than others. Among those who are less adaptable, there is a high degree of individual variation in terms of the specific balance of macronutrients that works best. The most effective way to find the balance that is right for you is to take a troubleshooting approach. If you are not having any running-related problems that may have a dietary link, stick with your current macronutrient balance and focus on upgrading the sources of your carbs, fats, and proteins. If you are having such a problem, make a targeted change and see if it helps. Following is a list of common running-related problems with a potential dietary link.

Problem	Possible Dietary Link
Low energy in workouts	Not enough carbohydrate
Unexpected fitness plateau	Not enough carbohydrate
Frequent illness	Not enough carbohydrate
Trouble shedding excess fat	Too much carbohydrate and/or too much fat
Lack of stride power	Not enough protein
Lingering muscle soreness	Not enough protein and/or fat
Frequent injuries	Not enough protein

HOW MUCH CARBOHYDRATE?

Nutrition experts who give dietary advice to athletes have been little affected by the so-called low-carb revolution. Almost without exception, these professionals still advise runners and other athletes to maintain a high-carbohydrate diet. Consequently, most runners continue to follow this advice, even as millions of their nonathletic peers scrupulously avoid fruit and other foods rich in sugars and starches. As mentioned earlier, the general recommendation is that runners get roughly 60 percent of their daily calories from carbohydrate. I don't think there's anything wrong with a diet that's 60 percent carbohydrate. But I also don't think there's anything wrong with a diet that's 40 percent, 50 percent, or even as much as 70 percent carbohydrate, as long as the carbohydrate is coming mostly from whole food sources.

The rationale behind the 60 percent recommendation is straightforward. Studies dating back several decades have shown that runners have better endurance when their muscles and liver are well stocked with glycogen. The more carbohydrate you consume on a daily basis, up to a point, the fuller your body's glycogen stores will be at any given time—hence the advice to eat lots of carbs. But the studies

THE RICHEST SOURCES

When properly balancing your macronutrients, it helps to know which foods are rich sources of each of the three macronutrients. Here are some examples. You can also learn the carbohydrate, fat, and protein content of foods by reading package labels, purchasing a book such as *The Complete Guide to Food Counts,* or by logging onto the USDA Nutrient Database at www.nal.usda.gov/fnic/foodcomp/search.

Carbohydrate-Rich Foods	Fat-Rich Foods	Protein-Rich Foods
Fruits	Deep ocean fish (e.g., haddock, cod, pollack)	Meats
Breakfast cereal	Olive oil	Poultry
Green, leafy vegetables	Nuts	Fish
Pasta	Vegetable oil	Soy
Rice	Milk and cheese	Nuts

proving the value of a glycogen-packed body have always done so in the context of a workout to complete exhaustion, wherein the orders are to go until you can go no more. While glycogen stores are indeed a major performance limiter in such extreme endurance tests, they are far less likely to be a performance limiter in everyday workouts, unless your diet is absurdly low in carbohydrates. So I don't think it's necessary to bring your glycogen stores back to the highest level possible after every workout. You can if you like, but a moderate-carbohydrate diet will do. And this is especially true if you consume 10 to 20 percent of your daily carbohydrate intake within an hour of completing each workout, as glycogen synthesis is at least twice as efficient within this window.

The results of a few studies have suggested that runners can perform at least as well in everyday training on a high-fat, moderate-carbohydrate diet as on a high-carbohydrate, low-fat diet. Other research has shown that most runners can adapt from either of these diet types to the other. In moving from a high-carb to a moderate-carb diet, runners initially experience a drop in performance, but after a few weeks their bodies adjust and their performance returns to normal.

This is good news for the many runners who do not respond well to a high-carbohydrate diet. These "carbohydrate-sensitive" individuals complain of fatigue, sluggishness, and poor running performance when they eat a high-carbohydrate diet. One of the runners I coach is carbohydrate-sensitive. He fares much better on the healthy moderate-carbohydrate diet he now maintains than he did on the high-carbohydrate diet he subjected himself to in the past.

It is also worth pointing out that, according to sports nutritionists, even runners who try to eat a high-carbohydrate diet often don't get as many carbs as they think. If you had your diet analyzed by a nutritionist, you might be as shocked by the discrepancy between how much carbohydrate you're actually eating versus how much you thought you were eating as I was when I had my diet analyzed. But don't consider this discrepancy a problem unless there is a problem with your health (such as trouble losing weight) or running (such as poor recovery from workouts). I'm confident that a majority of runners can do just fine on a diet ranging anywhere from 40 percent to 70 percent carbohydrate. Some runners will feel and perform best at the low end of this range, others toward the high end. I encourage you to experiment to find what works best for you.

The only time it really is important to maximize your body's glycogen stores is before long endurance tests, such as a marathon (or a run to exhaustion in a laboratory experiment!). But even then, the sort of crazed multi-day carbo-loading routine that was popular in the 1970s is hardly necessary. Remember, training greatly increases the muscles' general glycogen storage capacity, while individual workouts deplete these stores. Therefore, simply reducing your training volume (i.e., tapering) in the last several days before a longer race while eating as you normally do will swell your glycogen stores considerably. A simple, one-day carbo-loading protocol that I'll show you in Chapter 6 will top them off. If you then consume carbs regularly during the race, your muscles will have all the fuel they need for optimal performance.

HOW MUCH FAT?

The standard recommendation for dietary fat intake is no more than 30 percent of total calories. The nutrition experts who stand behind this recommendation believe that eating more fat causes health problems such as overweight and diabetes.

Athletes, including runners, are also frequently advised to keep their fat intake low to moderate (20 to 30 percent of calories) to leave plenty of room for carbs and protein, which are often considered more important to athletic performance.

However, research in general populations has shown that fat intake levels as high as 40 percent of total calories can be perfectly healthy. For example, one study found that European women who eat the most fat are the least likely to be obese. Likewise, research with runners and other athletes has shown that a high-fat diet does not adversely affect health or performance.

More important than the total amount of fat we consume is the balance of fats we consume. Our Paleolithic ancestors are believed to have eaten an even balance of saturated and unsaturated (i.e., mono- and polyunsaturated) fats. Today, the average American eats more than twice as much saturated fat as unsaturated fat. It is this type of imbalance that leads to health problems including obesity and heart disease. A high-fat diet in itself does not increase the risk for such conditions as long as the amount of saturated fat is not too high compared to the amount of unsaturated fat.

WHAT MAKES A MEAL?

This chart shows the carbohydrate, fat, and protein content of three typical meals (including a breakfast menu, a lunch menu, and a dinner menu).

	Carbohydrate	Fat	Protein
Granola with 2% milk	61%	42%	17%
Turkey sandwich with sprouts, lettuce, tomato, and mayonnaise	44%	34%	20%
Spaghetti with marinara sauce	67%	10%	22%

A recent analysis of the diet of elite Kenyan runners found that fat accounted for only 15 percent of their daily calories. So it's clear that a low-fat diet, while not necessary for good health and running performance, will not stand in the way of these things either. As with carbohydrate, there is a broad range of fat intake levels that can support optimal health and performance—anywhere from 15 to 40 percent of total calories. Some runners are able to function equally well on either a low-fat or a moderate-fat diet, while others feel best on one or the other. Again, you may need to experiment to discover what works best for you.

The one fat formula that applies to everyone is the ideal 1:1 ratio of saturated and unsaturated fats. Since most of us currently eat far more saturated fats than unsaturated fats, we need to reduce our consumption of the former and increase our consumption of the latter to find this balance. I'll say more about balancing fat types below.

HOW MUCH PROTEIN?

Protein is typically associated with strength athletes such as football players and bodybuilders. These athletes are interested in maximizing muscle force, which follows from increases in muscle size, which in turn results from protein accretion in the muscles. In fact, runners in heavy training require just as much protein, per pound of body weight, as football players and bodybuilders. While runners are not particularly interested in increasing the size of their muscles, they tend to experience higher levels of muscle protein degradation during training, so they need to consume extra protein just to keep their muscles functioning properly.

Scientists measure nitrogen balance—the amount of nitrogen entering the body in food versus the amount leaving the body in the urine—as an indirect way to measure whether muscles are growing or wasting. (Remember that nitrogen is present in all proteins but not in fats or carbohydrates.) When an athlete achieves a positive nitrogen balance, his or her muscles are almost certainly growing. Strength athletes seek to maintain what is called a state of positive nitrogen balance. Runners, on the other hand, simply want to avoid a negative nitrogen balance. Yet runners in heavy training need to consume protein in proportions equal to those that are recommended for strength athletes simply to avoid a deficit, the consequences of which include slower recovery from workouts, weaker adaptations to training, and increased risk of injury, illness, and overtraining. Even runners who maintain moderate training loads need to consume substantially more protein than the average person.

During running, muscle cells are damaged by oxygen radicals and also through mechanical stress. In addition, muscle proteins are broken down by catabolic hormones to provide a source of energy. When blood samples are taken from runners during long workouts and time trials, amino acids normally contained in muscle proteins are found to be present in extremely high levels—levels that are otherwise found only in people suffering from heart attacks and muscle-wasting diseases—indicating very high rates of muscle protein breakdown. These lost proteins must be replaced between workouts.

Having said all this, runners do not require more protein in the diet as a percentage of total caloric intake than nonathletes; they just require more total protein. This is true for fats and carbohydrates as well. Running increases the need for each of the macronutrients equally.

GOOD CARBS AND BAD CARBS

Ten years ago, few people had even heard of the glycemic index. Today, most health-conscious Americans know that the glycemic index is a measure of the rate at which blood glucose rises after a carbohydrate-containing food is eaten. Foods that provoke a strong glucose response are classified as high glycemic index (or high GI) foods; those that provoke a moderate glucose response are labeled moderate GI foods; and those that provoke a small glucose response are called low GI foods. Pure glucose (or sometimes white bread) is the reference "food," and is given a score of 100. Some examples of foods representing all three categories are given in the sidebar on page 62.

Conventional wisdom holds that high GI foods are unhealthy because they are essentially addictive, and overconsumption of such foods leads to weight gain, problems resulting from weight gain, and other negative health effects. The blood glucose surge following a high GI meal causes the pancreas to release large amounts of the hormone insulin, whose job it is to deliver glucose to various organs and tissues. But (so the theory goes) because very high blood glucose levels are toxic, the pancreas, somewhat panicked by the sudden glucose surge, releases more insulin than necessary, causing the blood glucose level to drop below normal (a phenomenon known as reactive hypoglycemia), triggering hunger and, specifically, cravings for more high GI foods.

Recent research has shown that reactive hypoglycemia is largely a myth, and that low blood glucose is not a significant physiological

HIGH, MODERATE, AND LOW GLYCEMIC FOODS

High Glycemic (>70)	Moderate Glycemic (55–70)	Low Glycemic (<55)
Baked potato (93)		
Corn flakes breakfast cereal (84)		
Gatorade (78)		
Ripe banana (77)		
Bagel (72)		
White rice (72)	Whole wheat bread (69)	
	Pineapple (66)	
	Ice cream (61)	
	Brown rice (55)	
	Green banana (55)	Old-fashioned oatmeal (49)
		Spaghetti (43)
		Peach (42)
		Snickers bar (41)
		Soybeans (41)

hunger trigger. In addition, there is no evidence that high GI foods are more likely to cause weight gain than moderate or low GI foods. Interestingly, the traditional Kenyan diet, and therefore the diet of many of the world's best runners, is extremely rich in high GI carbohydrates. The only real drawback of high GI carbohydrates is that they are not as long lasting an energy source as low GI carbohydrates. But there are times when runners need fast-acting carbohydrates. Before and during workouts and races, consuming high GI carbs such as those in sports drinks provides quick energy and enhances performance. A sports drink containing low GI carbohydrates would not supply fuel fast enough to help half as much. High GI carbs are also preferable immediately after exercise, when it's important to quickly replenish muscle and liver glycogen stores.

Many nutrition "experts" have taken to calling high GI carbs "bad carbs," but there is nothing inherently bad about high GI carbs. Bananas, raisins, and kidney beans are high GI foods. Nobody ever got fat or shortened his life span by eating bananas, raisins, and kidney beans. The only bad sources of carbohydrate are the highly processed ones, some of which are high GI, others of which are not. Foods containing refined grains that have been stripped of their fiber, vitamins, minerals, and phytonutrients are bad because they provide a lot of calories without a lot of other nutrition.

Also bad are foods that combine high amounts of carbohydrates and fats together. Such foods are almost nonexistent in nature. Outside of milk, nearly every food that is naturally high in fat is low in carbohydrate, and nearly every food that is naturally high in carbohydrate is naturally low in fat. But many processed foods (doughnuts, french fries, snack chips, etc.) are high in both carbohydrate and fat. Such foods are extremely calorie-dense (or energy-dense), meaning they pack a large number of calories in a small amount of space. This is a problem, because research has shown that people tend to eat a constant volume of food each day, regardless of how many calories are contained in that volume of food. So people who maintain a diet that is high in unnaturally calorie-dense foods are more likely to take in too many calories on a daily basis and develop an unhealthy body composition. To make matters worse, humans are naturally attracted to the taste and texture of foods that contain high amounts of fat and carbohydrate, so the temptation to give them a large place in the diet is great.

The best guideline to follow in selecting sources of carbohydrate is healthy eating principle #1: Eat natural foods. If you get the majority of your carbs from unprocessed or minimally processed sources such as fresh vegetables and whole grains, you will feel and perform better than if you get a lot of them from highly unnatural foods such as soft drinks and fried snack chips.

BALANCING YOUR FATS

As I suggested earlier, the problem with the typical American diet is not that it contains too much fat as a percentage of total calories but that it does not contain a good balance of fats. In particular, it contains too many saturated fats, too many trans fats and other damaged polyunsaturated fats, and not enough omega-3 essential fats. Eating too many saturated fats hardens arteries and cell membranes and has a variety of other negative consequences. Eating too few omega-3 essential fats diminishes the muscles' ability to recover from running-related tissue damage by compromising anti-inflammatory functions. Polyunsaturated fats that have been oxidized or otherwise damaged cause free radical damage in the body. And trans fats, as mentioned previously, are essentially poisonous.

Our Paleolithic ancestors consumed less saturated fat and more omega-3 fats than we do, and ate virtually no trans fats. Since the Paleolithic diet is the one our genes are best adapted to, it's important to balance our fats closer to the way these ancestors did (see the sidebar on page 65).

The most beneficial change you can make is to virtually eliminate trans fats from your diet. The best ways to reduce your intake of trans fats are to avoid fried foods and processed foods containing hydrogenated (or partially hydrogenated) oils. The main sources of oxidized polyunsaturated fats are bottled oils, which are bad not only because of this but also because such oils contain detergents, solvents, bleaches, and other toxins used in the refining process. Extra-virgin

IMPROVE THE BALANCE OF FATS IN YOUR DIET

Here are some simple strategies that will help you reduce your intake of saturated fats, trans fats, and damaged polyunsaturated fats and increase your intake of omega-3 fats.

Eat Less of These Foods . . .	**. . . And More of These**
Fried foods (high in trans and saturated fats)	Olive oil (low in damaged fats)
Processed foods containing "hydrogenated" or "partially hydrogenated" oils (high in trans fats and other damaged fats)	Fish oil and/or flax seed oil (high in omega-3s)
	Soybeans and soy foods (moderately high in omega-3s)
Fatty cuts of meat (high in saturated fats)	Raw nuts and seeds (high in undamaged polyunsaturated fats)
Whole milk dairy products (high in saturated fats)	Green leafy vegetables (moderately high in omega-3s)
All bottled cooking oils other than olive oil (high in damaged fats)	Low-fat dairy products (low in saturated fats)
Roasted nuts (high in damaged fats)	Organic meats and eggs (moderately high in omega-3s)

olive oil, which is produced without toxic chemicals and is low in polyunsaturated fats (hence naturally resistant to oxidation), is the only bottled oil you should use.

Saturated fats are often called "bad fats," but they are only bad in excess. They have many important roles in the body. Saturated fats are components of cell membranes that give them strength and stability. They protect the liver from toxins such as alcohol, facilitate the absorption of fat-soluble vitamins, and help the bones absorb calcium. And runners should be aware that they are the muscles' preferred fuel fat.

While it is common to think of saturated fats as the unhealthy fats in animal foods, every food that contains fat has saturated fats. For example, corn oil is 13 percent saturated fat, as is olive oil, and soybean oil is 16 percent saturated fat. It's true that animal foods contain more saturated fat than plant foods. This is largely because animals, humans included, *need* more saturated fat. Our adipose tissue, which is vital for energy storage, is almost all saturated fat.

On the other hand, there's a difference between needing something in the body and needing it in the diet. We are able to synthesize saturated fats in our bodies, which makes them nonessential in the diet. (They're almost impossible to avoid in the diet anyway.) Eating too much saturated fat does lead to less than optimal functioning and health, but no more than overeating any energy source does. It's just that saturated fats are a particularly common nutritional excess in our society. The average runner would benefit from reducing his or her saturated fat intake, because this will help improve the overall balance of fats in the diet.

Getting more omega-3 fats is easier said than done. Even if you eat more soy foods, fish, and meats produced from grass-fed animals, you may come up short some days, so I recommend taking a supplement. I'll say more about this later, and will return to the topic again in Chapter 9.

NOT ALL PROTEINS ARE THE SAME

Discussions about fats never fail to distinguish different types of fat that have different effects in the body. Likewise, discussions about carbohydrates never fail to distinguish different types of carbohydrate that have different effects in the body. But discussions about proteins almost always fail to explain that there are also different types of proteins that have different effects in the body.

The two most basic types of protein are animal proteins and plant proteins. There are some key differences between animal and plant

PROTEIN QUALITY

Scientists have various methods of measuring protein quality. Biological value (BV) is a measure of a particular protein's effect on nitrogen balance (the more positive the better). The protein digestibility-corrected amino acid score (PDCAAS) is a measure of how well a particular protein supplies the nine essential amino acids (the more completely the better). The following chart shows the BV and PDCAAS scores of several familiar protein sources, as well as the amount of protein each source contains in a typical portion.

	Biological Value	Protein Digestibility Corrected Amino Acid Score	Grams of Protein in a Typical Portion
Whole egg	100	1.00	6.5 (one egg)
Fish	82	0.8–0.92	41 (6 oz)
Beef	80	0.92	38 (6 oz)
Chicken	79	0.8–0.92	42 (6 oz)
Soy	74	0.91	10 (½ cup)
Peanuts	68	0.52	7.5 (1 oz)
Wheat	54	0.42	5 (2 slices whole wheat bread)

proteins from the perspective of those who eat them. First, animal proteins are more similar to human proteins than plant proteins are. For this reason, our bodies are able to make more efficient use of animal proteins. Second, unlike most animal proteins, most plant proteins contain very small amounts of, or are missing entirely, one or more of three essential amino acids: tryptophan, methionine, and lysine. This too makes plant proteins less effective in the body. Finally, animal foods tend to contain much larger amounts of protein than plant foods.

Clearly, animal foods provide higher-quality proteins and more of them. What is the practical significance of this fact? For nonathletes it makes no difference. They can easily get all the protein and all the essential amino acids they need by eating a well-balanced vegetarian diet. Athletes need more protein in general and, in particular, more of certain individual amino acids, including glutamine. A vegetarian runner can meet these needs with careful planning (I'll give nutrition strategies for vegetarian runners in Chapter 10), but a runner who includes at least some animal proteins in his or her diet can meet them much more easily, and it's possible that only a runner who includes at least some animal proteins in his or her diet can meet them optimally.

This is pure speculation on my part, as the effects of different protein types on running performance and recovery have not been studied. However, in some studies involving bodybuilders, diets that include animal proteins have resulted in significantly greater muscle mass gains than those that do not. The metabolic processes that allow runners to repair, remodel, and maintain their muscle tissues differ little from those that allow bodybuilders to gain muscle.

Because it is plausible that animal proteins are needed to achieve optimal performance nutrition, I recommend that you include wholesome sources of animal proteins in your diet unless you have a strong aversion to them, or ethical grounds for being vegetarian. If you are vegetarian, you can enhance your post-workout muscle repair and rebuilding by taking supplemental soy or whey protein after workouts. (Whey protein is derived from milk, so if you're vegan you'll have to use soy protein.)

IMPROVING ON NATURE

Natural foods are almost always the best sources for carbohydrates, proteins, and fats. However, there are some cases where processed sources of fats, proteins, and carbohydrates are preferable.

All in all, it's difficult to find unadulterated, natural sources of the essential omega-3 fatty acids. For this reason, take a daily oil supplement such as fish or flax oil, even though, as a processed food, it is an exception to the principle of eating natural foods. But not just any oil supplement will do. Because polyunsaturated oils are easily damaged by processing and oxidation, you have to choose your oil supplement very carefully. Your flax oil, for example, should be cold pressed, bought and kept in a refrigerated state, and contained in an opaque bottle, as even light can damage it. You should also buy it in small bottles to better your chances of using it up while it's still fresh.

As for carbohydrates and proteins, natural foods are definitely the best sources except within the "exercise interval"—that is, immediately before, during, and after workouts. At these times, no natural food can match the nutritional support for health, performance, and recovery that is offered by the ergogenic aids (sports drinks and energy gels) and recovery supplements that have been created especially for these uses. To begin with, you can't eat anything immediately before a run without getting an upset stomach during the run, and it's more or less impossible to eat solid food during a run. Water is beneficial immediately before and during a run, but it doesn't provide the electrolytes, carbohydrates, and in some cases protein or amino acids that a sports drink provides. Consequently, water, although more natural than a sports drink or energy gel, is significantly inferior with respect to hydration and energy supply.

After workouts, rapid provision of just the right nutrients has a major, positive impact on recovery. Performance recovery drinks such as Endurox R⁴ and Ultragen have been designed to deliver the ideal combination of nutrients more rapidly than any natural food. For example, both of the powdered drink mixes just mentioned contain whey protein isolate. Whey protein is one of two protein types found in milk (the other is casein). These two dairy proteins are separated from each other in the standard cheese-making process. Whey used to be considered a useless by-product of this process and was therefore discarded. However, when it was discovered that whey is actually a very high-quality protein, methods of distilling it into a powder containing little or no fat and lactose were developed and whey powder has since been used in a variety of protein supplements.

Whey protein is a complete protein that contains all nine essential amino acids. Its protein digestibility corrected amino acid score is 1.14, as compared to 0.94 for beef protein, and its biological value is an astronomical 149. In addition, whey protein empties from the stomach and is absorbed into the bloodstream from the intestine faster than other proteins. Therefore, supplements containing whey protein isolate—despite the fact that it is a processed protein—result in faster, better muscle recovery than natural foods.

Soy protein concentrate and soy protein isolate are proteins derived from soy. Although they are vegetable proteins, they are very high quality. In fact, a study conducted at The Ohio State University found that a soy protein supplement increased muscle mass in strength-training men as much as a whey protein supplement. There are a variety of protein and recovery supplements that use soy protein concentrate or isolate. If you're a vegan or strict vegetarian, you should use one after every workout.

CHAPTER 4

OPTIMIZING YOUR BODY COMPOSITION

According to the National Institutes for Health, more than a third of American women and nearly a quarter of American men are following some kind of weight loss diet at any given time. Among runners the figure is perhaps a little lower, but probably not by much.

The most popular means of pursuing weight loss are branded diet programs such as Weight Watchers. The various popular diets seem quite different on the surface, each claiming its own special reason for being more effective than the others. For example, the South Beach diet is supposed to facilitate weight loss by eliminating sugar cravings, while the so-called "fat flush diet" claims to shed fat pounds by detoxifying the liver. The truth is that all of the popular diets that are effective for some people (and most of them are effective for some people) share one reason for being so: significant calorie restriction.

A few years ago, the American Institute for Cancer Research (AICR) analyzed the diet plans in four successful diet books. None of the four plans promoted itself as a low-calorie diet. However, based on detailed analysis of each diet's specific portion recommendations, the AICR concluded that all four plans were essentially low-calorie diets. They just had different ways of restricting calories.

I believe that weight loss is not a worthy goal for most runners to pursue. A better alternative is to optimize your body composition—but not by dieting (severe calorie restriction). Research has shown that our health is affected not so much by how much we weigh, but rather by how lean we are—that is, by the ratio of fat-free mass to fat mass in our bodies (commonly measured as body fat percentage). Men and women who have a high body fat percentage tend to be unhealthy regardless of whether they are heavy or light. By contrast, individuals who have a low body fat percentage tend to be healthy, again regardless of whether they are heavy or light. The exceptions are those who have a very low body fat percentage *and* very low muscle weight, which indicates malnutrition/starvation. The healthiest men and women have good muscle tone and just enough body fat to perform the functions that body fat is responsible for, such as supplying energy.

A lean body composition is also ideal for athletic performance, because muscle is capable of performing work, whereas excess body fat just increases the load the muscles must carry. For these reasons, your weight is not the thing to be concerned about. It's your body composition that's important, with respect to both your overall health and your running. Of course, as a runner, there is an undeniable advantage to being light, but there's only so much you can do about that. Tall runners and large-framed runners cannot compete with shorter, small-framed runners for lightness. But any runner can achieve leanness and enjoy its benefits.

Optimizing body composition is different from simply losing weight. You can lose weight by losing fat, muscle, or even water. But to improve your body composition you must either lose fat or gain muscle, or do both. Many athletes feel they would perform better, not to mention look better, if they lost weight. But if you lose muscle (or water) instead of fat, your performance and health will only suffer. (Some heavily muscled individuals—usually men—can afford to lose some muscle mass if they want to transform themselves into distance runners.) And the method that people most often use to lose weight—general calorie restriction, or dieting—is sure to result in some muscle loss, and not necessarily much fat loss.

Severe calorie restriction not only doesn't optimize body composition (it wastes muscle along with fat), but it also compromises running performance by failing to provide adequate energy for workouts and recovery. Another problem with severe calorie restriction is that it's hard for people to sustain because it causes persistent hunger and requires followers to practice inhuman levels of self-denial of their favorite high-calorie foods. In a Tufts University study that investigated the effectiveness of four popular diets over the course of a year, more than half of the subjects dropped out before the study period was completed.

Specific popular diets cause additional problems for runners. Extreme low-carb diets, for example, rob the muscles of glycogen, their most important fuel, thereby causing running performance to plummet. What's more, since each gram of glycogen is stored along with 3 or 4 grams of water, extreme low-carb diets result in significant dehydration, which also wreaks havoc on running performance.

A much better way to optimize your body composition, especially as a runner, is to consume enough calories on a daily basis to sustain your optimal body composition. What does this mean? Imagine you have already achieved your optimal lean body composition and your goal is to keep it. The eating patterns required to do so are those that every runner should practice regardless of his or her current body composition. If you are currently above your personal optimal body fat percentage, whether by a little or a lot, you are probably consuming 1 to 5 percent more calories than would be necessary to maintain your optimal body fat level, supposing you were already there.

(I'll explain why in a moment.) By reducing your daily caloric intake just a little, you will—as long as you're exercising consistently—begin to slowly lose fat (and only fat) until you reach your ideal body composition. At this point, your body fat percentage will level off without you having to make any further adjustments to your diet.

This approach is very different from that of most popular diets, on which a person eats *less* than is required to support his or her ideal body composition to achieve rapid weight loss—with the drawbacks of constant hunger, muscle loss, and, for runners, compromised workout performance. Unlike dieting, eating for a very slight caloric deficit minimizes hunger and self-denial, ensures that you have enough energy to run well, and promotes fat loss over muscle loss.

Exercise itself is an essential complement to this approach to optimizing body composition. It improves the muscle mass to fat mass ratio by increasing muscle tone and by burning fat. Developing muscle tone through exercise also promotes leanness by increasing the resting metabolic rate—the rate at which your body burns calories at rest— as it costs more energy to sustain muscle than fat. And finally, a good running program reduces the caloric restriction required to achieve the negative caloric balance necessary to shed fat, making it even easier to keep hunger at bay without compromising your efforts.

Interestingly, daily exercise is the most widely shared habit among those who have successfully lost significant amounts of weight and kept it off for many years. Studies show that eating habits vary widely within this special population, but nearly all of its members exercise. That's a fact worth noting.

FOUR STEPS TO LEANNESS

It is natural to assume that people who are overweight, especially those who are severely overweight, eat far more calories than they need on a daily basis. This is seldom true. In fact, virtually no one maintains a large caloric surplus for any length of time. Even obese men and women typically eat less than 10 percent more calories per day than they need to meet their actual caloric needs (i.e., the amount of calories needed to sustain their optimal body composition). The reason is that our hunger and appetite are very well calibrated to our actual caloric needs. It's true that our hunger and appetite do tend to err on the side of caloric surplus, but by no more than a few percentage points in most of us. This is most likely because our appetite is calibrated to match the higher activity level that was the norm during our evolutionary development.

Even a tiny surplus can lead to significant fat storage and weight gain over many years. For example, a 150-pound runner who eats 100 calories a day more than he needs, a mere 4 percent surplus, will gain approximately 10 pounds of body fat in a year. The good news is that because very few of us maintain a caloric surplus of more than a few percentage points, it's possible to create the slight caloric deficit you need to improve your body composition by making just a few small dietary changes and running consistently. The number of daily calories you need to achieve this goal is probably only 3 to 5 percent less than you currently consume—assuming your body fat percentage is worse than ideal.

Although there's no formula to determine your optimal body composition, for the purpose of the following example, we'll pretend there is. Suppose that, to reach your optimal body composition, you would need to weigh 150 pounds. As a runner you would need to eat about 2,550 calories a day to sustain this body composition. This is the amount of energy you should consume regardless of your actual weight. But let's say your current weight is 175 pounds. If this is the case, you are probably consuming roughly 2,700 calories per day. So all you need to do to optimize your body composition is trim 150 calories per day from your diet—or approximately the number of calories in one serving of potato chips. As you can see, even though you're carrying 25 pounds of excess body fat (in this hypothetical example!), a very small caloric reduction will get rid of it.

Maintaining a slight caloric deficit does not require calorie counting, and in fact calorie counting does not really work for this purpose because the methods are too approximate. Guides such as *The Complete Book of Food Counts* by Corinne T. Netzer allow you to roughly estimate your daily caloric intake. They tell you how many calories are contained in a single serving of everything you eat and drink in a day. You then have to measure or estimate the amount of each food type (i.e., the number of servings) you eat and add it all together. At the same time, you can use any one of various calculators to determine your basal metabolic rate (BMR), which is the number of calories your body uses just to keep you alive for 24 hours, and also to determine how many extra calories you burn through activities ranging from working at a desk to running. To estimate the total number of calories burned in a day, you have to add your BMR and the extra calories burned through all activities more vigorous than lying still. This is a lot of work, and studies of these methods have shown that they are too approximate to accurately pinpoint the combination of activity and food intake required to achieve a modest caloric deficit. The difference between a small caloric deficit and small caloric surplus could be as little as 2 percent—well within the margin of error of these methods of estimation.

Instead of counting calories, follow a simple four-point plan to optimize your body composition.

1. Measure your body fat percentage to establish a starting point.
2. Make targeted changes to your diet and other lifestyle habits that will improve your body composition.

3. Measure your body fat percentage regularly to track your progress.

4. Monitor your running as a check against becoming too lean or making changes that are not beneficial to your well-being (as anything that harms your health will harm your running, too).

Measuring your body fat allows you to pursue the goal of improving it objectively. Two testing methods are relatively inexpensive and convenient. One option is to have a nutritionist or personal trainer estimate your body fat percentage using a plastic caliper to take skin-fold measurements. This will cost you between $25 and $50 per test.

A second option is to purchase a body fat tester for home use, such as the Omron HB-306. These devices use bioelectrical impedance to estimate body composition with reasonable accuracy. Expect to pay about $60 for one of these devices, which are available through many exercise equipment retailers. The advantage of self-testing is that you can do it whenever you want.

The American Council on Exercise offers the following guidelines for body fat percentage in men and women:

	Men	Women
Essential fat	2–4%	10–12%
Athletic range	6–13%	14–20%
Fitness range	14–17%	21–24%
Acceptable range	18–25%	25–31%

Once you have determined your current body composition, set incremental goals to improve it. If you are currently above the acceptable range, set a modest initial goal of moving down into it. If you're currently in the middle of the acceptable range, set a goal of moving down into the fitness range. Don't automatically aim straight for the bottom of the athletic range. Not everyone can get there safely, and no one gets there overnight. Focus on the *means* of improving body composition—smart training and proper nutrition—and the numbers will take care of themselves.

I recommend testing your body composition once every 2 weeks. To ensure maximum accuracy using this method, conduct the measurements under the same circumstances each time: for example, first thing in the morning every other Saturday. Don't expect to see progress every time you measure—it's the overall trend that's important.

Of course, it's possible that your first body fat test will reveal that you already have an athletic body fat percentage, which means you are probably already eating to sustain your optimal body composition. In this case, continued testing will only serve to keep you on track. But even if your body fat percentage is low already, you should begin to practice any and all of the 21 ways to optimize your body composition given in the next section that are not already habits in your life. They are healthy habits for anyone, so even if they don't make you leaner, they still might make you healthier and enhance your running.

Is it possible that your body fat percentage could fall too low? Except in cases of disordered eating this does not happen often, but it can happen. Your safeguard against losing too much body fat is your running performance. If your body fat should ever fall to an unhealthy level, your running will begin to suffer. As long as you are running well—feeling consistently strong in your workouts and recovering quickly after them—you can trust that you have enough body fat to do its job.

Every man and woman, regardless of his or her body fat percentage—whether way too high, slightly too high, optimal, or even too low—should eat as if his or her body composition were already ideal and the goal was to sustain it. And the same means apply to everyone as well: train smart, obey the four principles of healthy eating, measure your body fat consistently, tweak your diet to move your body fat percentage in the right direction, and monitor your running performance as a way to safeguard against going too far in either direction.

STRATEGIES FOR IMPROVED BODY COMPOSITION

The following are small but effective strategies for tweaking your eating patterns to reduce caloric intake, or to make better use of the calories you're already taking in. Some will also enhance the quality of your training to help you get leaner as a by-product of improved running fitness.

Replace beverages with water. The calories contained in beverages such as soft drinks and fruit juices can really add up. Replacing some or all of these drinks with water is an easy way to eliminate dozens of calories from your daily intake. For example, a 12-ounce can of Pepsi contains 150 calories. Water, of course, has none.

Make one exception for sports drinks used during running. Although sports drinks do contain a lot of calories, these calories help you run at a higher level, and by doing your workouts at a higher performance level you will improve your body composition.

Eat breakfast. A spate of recent research has shown that *when* we eat is almost as important as *what* we eat with respect to optimizing our body composition. Nutrition scientists have learned that it's essential to coordinate energy intake with energy expenditure throughout the day. Calories are put to their best possible use when they are consumed at times when there is a strong demand for them in the body.

Morning is a time of relatively high caloric demand, as the body has gone 8 to 12 hours without any nutrition by the time the alarm clock sounds. Meeting the body's morning caloric needs by eating breakfast has been shown to reduce caloric intake later in the day. It may also increase your activity level by providing more energy in the morning. The net result is fewer total calories consumed and more total calories burned over the course of the entire day. A study from the University of Massachusetts found that those who regularly skip breakfast are 4.5 times more likely to be overweight than those who eat it most mornings.

Graze. Eating smaller meals more frequently (5 or 6 times a day) is another proven way to better coordinate food intake with energy needs. A study published in the *British Medical Journal* found that those who ate most frequently were thinner and had lower cholesterol and triglyceride levels than those who ate least often. As with eating breakfast, the reason seems to be that more frequent eating reduces appetite and increases activity levels.

Eat smaller portions. There is evidence that average food portion sizes have increased over the past few decades. We are served larger portions in restaurants, and we are also loading our plates and bowls more heavily when serving ourselves at home. In one long-term study, portion control was shown to be the most effective tool for weight loss. Simply serve yourself slightly smaller portions than you are accustomed to eating. Don't worry about going hungry. Remember, your goal is to reduce your total daily caloric intake by just a few percentage points, so you need only trim your portion sizes by a similar amount.

Fuel your workouts properly. Perhaps the gravest nutrition mistake runners make when pursuing weight loss is to avoid taking in nutrition before and during workouts for fear of "nullifying" the calorie-burning effect of the workout. Nothing could be further from the truth. Runners who do not fuel their workouts properly by consuming an adequate pre-workout meal and either a sports drink or energy gels plus water during runs inevitably consume an equal number of calories in other forms later in the day. It is preferable to use those calories to fuel a good workout, because the better you perform in your workouts, the stronger will be the various training effects you derive from them—and this includes improvements in body composition.

Fuel your recovery properly. During times of heavy training, many endurance athletes have difficulty maintaining muscle mass. Consistently taking in proper nutrition immediately after workouts makes it a lot easier. Remember that losing muscle mass worsens body composition no less than gaining fat does.

The most important recovery nutrients are carbohydrate and protein, and it is equally crucial that these nutrients be consumed as soon as possible after training. This was demonstrated indirectly in a study published in the *Journal of Physiology*. Subjects were given a carbohydrate-protein supplement either immediately after exercise or 2 hours later while participating in a 12-week strength-training program. In subjects receiving a carbohydrate-protein mixture immediately after each exercise session, muscle size increased 8 percent and strength improved 15 percent. When the supplement was given 2 hours later, there was no muscle growth or improvement in strength. Although runners are seldom interested in gaining muscle, these results are equally relevant to the goal of simply preserving muscle.

Proper recovery nutrition may reduce body fat levels while preserving or increasing lean muscle mass. Using laboratory animals, Japanese researchers were the first to investigate the cumulative effects of recovery nutrition on both muscle mass and body fat. For 12 weeks they fed rats either immediately after exercise or 4 hours later. After 12 weeks, muscle weight was 6 percent higher and abdominal fat 24 percent lower in the rats fed immediately. It is almost certain that the effects of proper recovery nutrition on the body composition of humans are similar.

Cut back on "sin" foods. Foods containing large amounts of sugar (e.g., desserts) and/or saturated or trans fats (e.g., french fries) cannot have a large place in your diet if you wish to optimize your body composition. On the other hand, you don't need to eliminate these foods entirely, and if you tend to crave them, you definitely should not try to eliminate them. Completely denying yourself your favorite treats can be rather unpleasant, and all too often those who attempt it wind up "snapping" and binging on them, which is worse than keeping them in the diet but shrinking their place in it. For example, if you like to have something sweet after dinner, and your present habit is to eat a big bowl of ice cream, try replacing it with a single chocolate candy. I did this very thing and it has worked out splendidly. A chocolate candy has about 200 fewer calories than a bowl of ice cream, yet it satisfies my dessert craving just as well.

Be more consistent. Healthy eating is not like a vaccine: one shot and you're covered for life. Instead, it requires a daily, life-long commitment. There is evidence that the more consistent you are in your wholesome eating habits, the greater your chances of maintaining a healthy body weight.

The National Weight Control Registry (NWCR) is a pool of research subjects comprising several thousand men and women who have lost an average of 66 pounds apiece and kept the weight off for an average of 6 years. For a number of years, scientists have been studying the habits of these subjects in search of the keys to successful weight loss maintenance. One of the most recent findings is that people who successfully lose weight maintain a very consistent eating pattern from day to day and throughout the year. Unlike many dieters, they tend to eat the same during the workweek as on the weekends. They also eat consistently throughout the year, engaging in less holiday indulgence than the average person. Follow their example.

Eat out less often. According to the results of a study performed by researchers at Tufts University, adults who eat frequently at restaurants are significantly fatter than those who dine out less often. This is because we tend to eat larger portions and less balanced meals in restaurants. If you eat out frequently, try replacing at least one or two restaurant meals with healthy meals eaten or prepared at home. You'll not only cut calories, you'll also save money.

For a busy person who doesn't enjoy cooking—and that probably describes most of us—this habit can be hard to change. But by taking it slowly, learning simple recipes that are healthy and tasty, one by one, you can achieve great overall results in time. Boil some rice. Slice up some chicken breasts, peppers, and zucchini. Sauté them in a skillet with olive oil and teriyaki sauce. Toss the meat and vegetables over the rice. You just cooked!

Redefine "full." Many of us have a habit of stuffing ourselves at meals, without being conscious of it. We have fallen into relying on a skewed definition of "fullness" that promotes overeating. Give fullness (nutritionists call it satiety) a healthier definition by using a 1-to-5 scale of fullness to determine when you should stop eating at meals. If 5 equals "stuffed," stop eating at 3 or 4, when you are comfortably full instead of uncomfortably so.

"But," you ask, "won't this result in my becoming hungry again sooner?" It might, but remember, most of us don't eat often enough anyway, and we tend to eat fewer calories overall when our meals are smaller and more frequent. What's more, even if it does not decrease your total daily caloric intake, reducing the size of your meals may decrease the number of calories you wind up storing as fat. This is because large meals containing far more carbohydrate and/or fat calories than are needed to meet your immediate energy needs result in large amounts of fat storage, whereas smaller meals that supply just enough calories to meet short-term energy needs result in minimal fat storage.

Get more sleep. Sleep deprivation increases levels of the hormone grehlin, which stimulates appetite and decreases levels of leptin, a hormone that suppresses appetite. According to one study, those who get only 2 to 4 hours of sleep per night are 73 percent more likely to be obese than those who sleep 7 to 9 hours. Individual sleep needs vary, but most people need 7 to 9 hours. The average adult sleeps slightly less than 7 hours per night. If you're even slightly sleep deprived on a chronic basis, do something about it, and you will be well rewarded with less hunger, not to mention a host of other benefits ranging from increased productivity to fewer illnesses.

Pay attention. Research has shown that simply paying attention to what you eat is one of the more effective ways to reduce your caloric intake. Self-monitoring strategies are a key habit among members of the NWCR. About half of them report that they still count calories and fat grams even years after their initial weight loss. Again, it's not necessary to count every single calorie you put in your mouth, but it is helpful to read food labels, pay attention to portion sizes, and generally be aware of what and how much you eat and drink throughout the day. As mentioned previously, keeping a food journal for at least a few days is a good way to become more aware of your true eating patterns. Research has found that there is a consistent gap between people's beliefs about their diet and the reality.

Another useful self-monitoring habit that is also used by most members of the NWCR is keeping track of your weight. It's a good idea to hop on the scale once a week even after you've attained your desired body composition because doing so will help you avoid the insidious upward creep that is the undoing of many initially successful diets. With frequent weigh-ins you can catch an upward trend very early and make adjustments to nip it in the bud. Continuing to check your body composition every couple of weeks or so is useful in this regard as well.

Get back on the horse. Most diets come to an end when the dieter cheats for a day or two or gains a pound or two and then abruptly decides that it's pointless to continue. This is a little like abandoning a marathon training program due to an illness that forces you to miss just a couple of workouts. Setbacks and slipups are inevitable in any healthy eating program. Understanding the importance of staying consistent can minimize setbacks and slipups, but it won't eliminate them. That's not a problem. The problem is allowing these inevitable situations to destroy your morale, as people all too often do. Even if you eat poorly for a whole week, it's not too late to get back on track. Within another 2 or 3 weeks, those 7 days of dietary backsliding will appear as nothing more than a speed bump.

Eliminate "screen eating." For many of us, the difference between a slight caloric deficit and a slight caloric surplus is the unconscious snacking we do in front of TV and computer screens. If you have a screen eating habit, you might want to institute a rule forbidding it. While somewhat gimmicky, this small prohibition can be effective for some. It's no accident that, according to research, those who watch the most television are also the most likely to be overweight.

Spoil your appetite. Have you ever thought about what makes you feel full after eating a meal? It's a special hormone called cholecystokinin

(CCK). When protein and fat from a meal begin to empty from the stomach, the small intestine releases CCK, which does three important things: It slows the emptying of food from the stomach; it stimulates nerves in the stomach, which tell the brain that the stomach is full; and it travels to the brain, where it acts on specific CCK receptors in the appetite control center. The net result is that you begin to feel full and lose interest in eating. After you finish eating, your body activates mechanisms that turn off CCK so you can become hungry again.

You can "trick" this mechanism to the advantage of your efforts to optimize your body composition by eating a small snack containing protein and/or fat about 20 minutes before a meal. By the time you sit down, the level of CCK in your blood will be rising and you'll eat a smaller meal. Examples of low-calorie appetite spoilers are three or four celery sticks dipped in peanut butter, three or four crackers with cheese, and two or three low-fat mozzarella cheese sticks.

There are also some over-the-counter products designed specifically to spoil your appetite before meals by stimulating CCK. The advantage of these products—called satiety aids—over regular foods is that they stimulate more CCK with fewer calories. One such product is Be Lean, which are chocolate-flavored chews whose active ingredient is glycomacropeptide, a natural product of soy digestion that also happens to be an especially powerful CCK stimulator. One study showed that eating a product similar to Be Lean reduced the size of a subsequent meal by 20 percent.

Eat filling foods. The concept of caloric density, or energy density, refers to the number of calories per unit volume in a given food. A food that packs a lot of calories in a small area is said to have high caloric density. Because water and dietary fiber are, for the most part, noncaloric, foods that contain a lot of water and/or fiber tend to have low caloric density. Processed foods tend to be calorically dense, while fruits and vegetables, with their high water and fiber content, are less dense.

Caloric density is important for those seeking to optimize their body composition because research has shown that people tend to eat a consistent volume of food regardless of the number of calories it contains. This was demonstrated in a Penn State study in which women were fed either a high-density, medium-density, or low-density meal three times a day. All participants received instructions to eat as much as they wanted. The subjects in all three groups ate the same *weight* of food, but the women eating the high-density meals took in 30 percent more calories than the women eating the low-density meals.

The lunch entrée, for example, was a pasta bake made from pasta shells, zucchini, broccoli, carrots, onions, tomato sauce, and parmesan, mozzarella, and ricotta cheeses. The low-density version contained more vegetables, while the medium- and high-density versions contained more shells and cheese. This example demonstrates how you can reduce your daily caloric intake in general without "eating less." Just reduce the amount of high-fat and refined-carb foods and increase the amount of fruits and vegetables.

Make it a team effort. Losing fat alone is harder than losing fat with a buddy or significant other. In a recent study at the University of Pittsburgh, subjects who enrolled in a clinical weight loss program with family or friends were 19 percent more likely to complete the program, lost more weight, and were three times as likely to maintain their weight loss as those who enrolled alone. Encourage your spouse or significant other to join you in your healthy eating project. The moral support and practical help you can provide each other will greatly increase your chances of sticking with it. If you live alone, make a healthy eating pact with a friend such as a running partner.

Tackle stress. Recently the effects of stress on weight gain have been a hot research topic. It is well established now that stress hormones, particularly cortisol, do promote fat storage and resist fat burning. Stress is also linked to a long list of other health problems, so its role in overweight is just one more reason to make every effort to reduce the amount of stress in your life.

There are many ways to reduce both the causes of stress and the severity of the physiological response with which your body reacts to these stressors. I will share several stress reduction strategies in Chapter 7.

Train consistently. Some runners allow themselves to get rather out of shape over the winter. You don't have to—and in most cases shouldn't—train as hard over the winter as you do during the summer, but it's best to stay consistently active year-round to avoid holiday weight gain. Research has shown that most weight gain occurs during the winter, and that most winter weight gain is never lost. So if you need a break from running at this time, don't go cold turkey on working out, but instead go for alternatives such as swimming, strength training, and cross-country skiing.

Train progressively. Failure to train progressively is one of the most common mistakes runners make. In order to achieve maximum fitness for your next big race, your training should be divided into three phases designed to build your fitness toward a peak that is timed to coincide with an important race.

Phase one is the base phase of training. The objective of base phase training is to develop the ability to handle a high overall volume of running and to handle some challenging high-intensity workouts during the subsequent build phase without breaking down. This is achieved by performing a gradually increasing volume of mostly moderate-intensity running, plus a small amount of very high-intensity running and some appropriate cross-training (especially for strength). As a general rule, and up to a point, the more easy running you do in the base phase, the more hard running you can do later.

In the second phase of training, called the build phase, the objective is to build on your fitness base to create a surplus of the speed and endurance adaptations you're looking for. Finally, during the peak phase, you integrate these adaptations by emphasizing workouts that are performed at or near race pace.

Within each phase, make your training progressive by making your key workouts (your hardest and longest runs) more and more challenging. For example, in your first tempo run (see below), do just 20 minutes. In the following week's tempo run, do 22 minutes, then 24 minutes, and so on.

Vary your training. Another common training mistake is insufficient workout variation. The bread-and-butter workout of many runners is a steady run of medium duration at a moderate intensity. There is nothing inherently wrong with this type of run, which I call a foundation run, but there are several other types of running workouts that you should also do because they affect your fitness in different ways. And remember, anything you do that positively affects your running fitness will also positively affect your body composition. Following are brief descriptions of seven basic workout types that belong in every runner's program:

Recovery runs are short (20 to 45 minutes), steady runs performed at a very easy intensity. Your next run following a hard run such as an intervals workout should usually be a recovery run. These quick and easy runs allow you to do more total running than you could if you ran hard all the time, and they also allow you to run harder in your workouts that are supposed to be hard.

Foundation runs are medium-duration (30 to 90 minutes), steady runs performed at a comfortable pace. Most of the runs you do in the early part of the training process (called the base phase) should be of this type. However, in the latter part of the training process these should give way to more challenging workouts and recovery runs. Foundation runs build aerobic capacity and the ability of the musculoskeletal system to handle repetitive impact.

Long runs are extended foundation runs. "Long" is a relative term. What counts as long in training for 5K races might not qualify as long in a marathon training program, and what counts as long for you in the base phase of training might no longer qualify as long near the end of the program. The main purpose of long runs is to enhance endurance.

Tempo runs are 20 to 40 minutes of steady running at a pace that's a little slower than your 10K race pace, sandwiched between a thorough warmup and cooldown (easy jogging and perhaps some stretching). After completing the base phase of training you should do tempo runs once a week. Their purpose is to increase the maximum pace you are able to maintain for a prolonged duration.

Interval workouts consist of short segments of hard running separated by segments of recovery jogging. Interval workouts should always begin with a thorough warmup and end with a cooldown. Short intervals (200 to 600 meters) increase aerobic capacity and running economy and are best suited to the middle period of the training process (the build phase). Longer intervals (800 to 1600 meters) increase resistance to neuromotor fatigue (that burning feeling in your legs!) and are best suited to the final, peak phase of training.

Intervals are generally run on a track.

Fartlek runs are interval workouts performed in an off-road environment. They achieve the same effects, but some runners (those who don't like running in circles) find them more enjoyable.

Hill workouts are short-interval workouts wherein the segments of hard running are performed on a moderate incline. The best time to do hill workouts is in the late base phase and/or early build phase, in order to transform the general strength you've built through strength training (see below) into more run-specific strength.

Strength train. Every runner should engage in regular strength training, because doing so has been proven to prevent a variety of injuries and enhance running performance. Strength training prevents injuries primarily by enhancing joint stability. Inadequate joint stability, especially in the knees, hips, and pelvis, is a major cause of many of the most common running injuries.

Strength training enhances running performance by increasing stride power—that is, the force with which a runner is able to push off the ground with each stride. In a Swedish study, trained runners replaced 32 percent of their running with plyometrics (jumping drills). After 9 weeks, their maximum sprint speed, running economy, and 5K race times improved.

A side benefit of strength training, for runners trying to improve their body composition, is that the muscle development resulting from strength training helps burn off body fat by raising the resting metabolic rate.

Many runners are reluctant to strength train because they fear they will gain weight. But research shows this won't happen if you also get regular cardiovascular exercise.

Following is a basic strength workout for runners. Start with one set of each exercise and build up to three sets performed in a circuit (i.e., do one set of each exercise, then a second set of each, etc.). Do the workout two times a week during periods when you are racing or training toward a race and three times a week at other times.

STICK CRUNCH

Lie on your back, bend your knees, and draw them as close to your chest as possible. Grasp any type of stick or rod (such as a broom handle) with both hands, positioned shoulder width apart. Begin with your arms extended straight toward your toes (A). Now squeeze your abdominal muscles and reach forward with the stick until it passes beyond your toes (B). Pause for 1 second and relax. Do 15 to 30 repetitions.

Benefit: This situp variation strengthens the abdominal wall and improves the stability of the pelvis and lower spine during running.

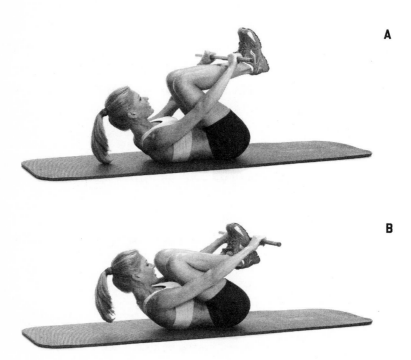

A

B

SIDE STEPUP

Stand about 1 foot to the left of a 12- to 18-inch platform (such as an exercise bench) with your right foot resting flat on this support and your left foot on the floor, so that your right knee is moderately bent and your left leg is straight (A). Shift your weight onto your right foot and straighten your right leg, raising your whole body upward (B). Pause briefly with your left foot suspended next to your right foot and then bend your right leg again, lowering your left foot back to the floor. Do 10 to 12 repetitions, then switch legs. For a greater challenge, do this exercise with a weighted barbell braced on your upper back or holding dumbbells in your hands.

Benefit: This exercise strengthens the thighs, hips, and glutes, improving knee and hip stability.

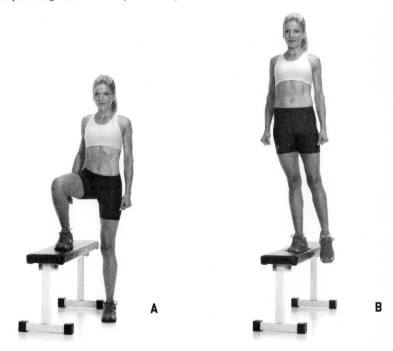

A   B

PILLOW BALANCING

Remove your shoes, place a pillow on the floor, and balance on it with one foot for 30 seconds. Then balance on the other foot and repeat. At first it will be difficult to last 30 seconds, but you'll quickly improve. Keep it challenging by using a bigger or softer pillow, by stacking pillows, and/or by balancing longer.

Benefit: This improves ankle stability by strengthening the muscles that oppose the calf muscles.

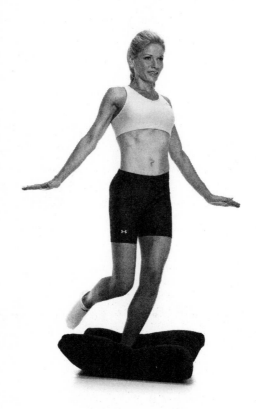

HIP TWIST

Lie face up with your arms resting out to your sides and your palms flat on the floor. Extend your legs directly toward the ceiling, keeping your feet together, and point your toes (A). Keeping your big toes side-by-side, tip your legs 12 to 18 inches to the right by twisting at the hip, so that your left buttock comes off the floor (B). Fight the pull of gravity by maintaining stability with your abs and obliques. Pause for a moment, then return slowly to the start position, again using your core muscles to control the movement. Repeat on the left side. Do 8 to 12 repetitions on each side.

· ·

Benefit: This exercise strengthens the abdominal muscles, including the obliques, improving pelvic stability.

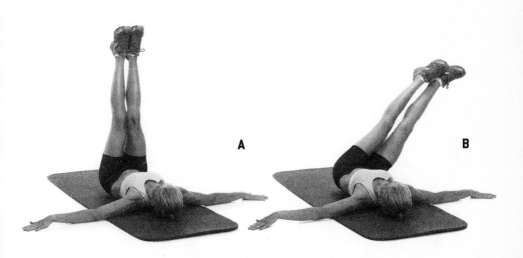

A   B

SINGLE ARM DUMBBELL SNATCH

Assume a wide athletic stance with a single dumbbell placed on the floor between your feet. Begin with your left arm fully extended and bend forward from the hips and grasp the dumbbell with your left hand (A). With a single, fluid, powerful movement, pull the dumbbell off the floor, stand fully upright, and continue raising your left arm until it is extended straight overhead (B). Pause briefly and then reverse the movement, allowing the dumbbell to come to rest again on the floor briefly before initiating the next lift. Complete 10 to 12 repetitions and then switch to the right arm.

Benefit: Strengthens the thighs, hips, glutes, lower and upper back, chest, and shoulders, improving knee and hip stability and running posture.

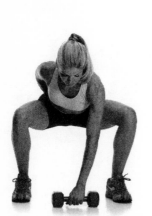

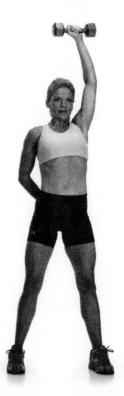

A

B

CHAPTER 5

HYDRATION AND NUTRITION DURING RUNNING

In the sport of distance running today, the most problematic illegal performance-enhancing substances are recombinant erythropoietin (rEPO) and anabolic androgenic steroids. A century ago it was water. Believe it or not, until the second half of the twentieth century, drinking during races was widely considered to be unsportsmanlike, if not outright cheating. Many runners also considered it a sign of weakness. The prevailing mentality held that the fitter and tougher the runner, the longer he could go in a workout or race without giving in to his thirst. (I say "he" and "his" because there were very few female distance runners during the first several decades of the sport's modern era, which dates from the late nineteenth century.) Consequently, in the old days, runners customarily avoided drinking while running.

Paradoxically, many of the same runners who believed that water offered an "unfair" advantage also believed that drinking while running was harmful to performance, and eschewed it for this reason as well. While recognizing the benefits of water with respect to body hydration, these runners were convinced that the cramping, bloating, and uncomfortable sloshing that it sometimes caused were too high a price to pay. Only when science was able to prove that dehydration was not only bad for performance but also potentially dangerous did attitudes and practices begin to change. In 1977, in reaction to this evidence, the International Amateur Athletic Federation finally relaxed regulations that until then had strictly limited allowable fluid intake during long-distance races.

By this time, a physician named Robert Cade at the University of Florida had created the first sports drink. Cade hypothesized that the addition of electrolyte minerals and carbohydrates to water would facilitate fluid replacement and provide an energy source to working muscles, thereby enhancing athletic performance and delaying fatigue better than water alone could do. He named the drink Gatorade, because it was first used by the Florida "Gators" football team.

Cade and other researchers tried various concentrations and carbohydrate combinations until they settled on a basic formula that maximized the rate of gastrointestinal absorption. This was important, because it resulted in faster delivery of nutrients to the blood and working muscles and minimized some of the classic gastrointestinal problems that were commonly associated with trying to drink on the run. Clinical trials of this revolutionary new sports fuel confirmed that it did indeed enhance athletic performance and delay fatigue better than plain water.

For this reason—and for several other reasons that I cite below—I believe that runners should use a good sports drink during most workouts and all longer races. Unfortunately, despite all we've learned in the past 50 years, most runners still drink nothing at all during the majority of their workouts and are as likely to drink water as anything else when they do drink. In my experience, the situation in which many runners are most likely to drink on the run is, ironically, during short to middle-length races (5K, 10K, etc.)—one of the few situations in which drinking anything does more harm than good. The objective of this chapter is to help you bring your hydration and nutrition practices during running into the twenty-first century, once and for all.

THE MANY BENEFITS OF SPORTS DRINKS

Quick: Name five benefits of using a sports drink during workouts and races. If you're like most athletes, you can only name one or two. The benefit all athletes know about is hydration. Or do they? More than 30 years after Gatorade first hit the market, television commercials for the original sports drink are still driving home the point that it "hydrates better than water," which I take as a sign that this remains news to many.

A second benefit of sports drinks that at least most runners know about (if not other athletes) is energy. Sports drinks contain carbohydrates, and carbohydrates are the body's preferred energy source during intense activity.

Are there really three more benefits of sports drinks? Actually, there are now no fewer than seven proven benefits, which together should motivate you to make a good sports drink part of your daily training.

BENEFIT #1: BETTER HYDRATION

Perspiration is a vital cooling mechanism for the body. Almost three-quarters of the energy that working muscles release during running takes the form of heat waste. If this heat were allowed to accumulate in the muscles it would cause serious tissue damage. The blood carries some of the excess heat away from the muscles to capillaries near the surface of the skin. Sweat glands then take up some fluid from the blood, and with it some heat, and release it onto the surface of the skin where it evaporates. Finally, cooled blood flows back toward the core of the body to absorb and distribute more heat. The only problem with this mechanism is that it's essentially self-sabotaging. The more you sweat, the more your blood volume shrinks, and the more your blood volume shrinks, the less heat your circulation can carry away from the working muscles, and the less effective perspiration becomes.

Runners often produce sweat at rates exceeding 1.5 liters per hour. About 10 percent of this fluid comes from water released when glycogen (the storage form of glucose in the muscles) is metabolized. Since this water serves no other function than assisting glycogen storage, its loss does no harm. But about 90 percent of sweat comes directly from the blood. Drinking while running can slow dehydration substantially. It can't stop it, though, because the average runner is unable to tolerate drinking more than 500 to 700 milliliters per hour at moderate running intensities. Drinking any faster causes uncomfortable stomach sloshing and can eventually result in cramps, bloating, and nausea.

As already mentioned, sports drinks hydrate better than water. Why? Three reasons: First, fluids are absorbed through the gut and into the bloodstream faster when their osmolality closely matches that of the blood itself. Osmolality is the concentration of dissolved particles in a fluid. Sports drinks contain dissolved minerals (sodium, etc.) and carbohydrates, as does the blood itself, whereas water contains only trace amounts of various dissolved minerals and elements, so the latter can't reach the bloodstream as quickly.

Sodium and other minerals also play important roles in regulating fluid balance in the body. In other words, they help determine how much fluid enters muscle fibers and other cells, how much remains in the blood, and so forth. Because sports drinks contain these minerals, they do a better job of allowing the body to maintain optimal fluid balance, which is an important aspect of hydration status. (It's not just *how much* fluid is in your body that matters, but *where it is*.)

A third advantage of sports drinks over water with respect to hydration is that the sodium content of sports drinks stimulates thirst, so athletes usually drink more when they have a sports drink than when they have plain water.

Under most circumstances, consuming water is better than drinking nothing, but not always. During workouts and races that last 4 hours or more, "replacing" sweat with only plain water can result in a dangerous dilution of the blood. Hyponatremia, or water intoxication, is a potentially deadly condition that results when the sodium concentration of the blood falls too low due to prolonged sweating combined with excessive water intake. Symptoms include dizziness, muscle cramping, confusion, and stomach bloating. Severe cases can lead to seizure, coma, and even death.

Hyponatremia occurs most often during marathons, when runners are running longer and drinking more (water) than at just about any other time. Noncompetitive runners who require more than 4 hours to complete a marathon are most susceptible to hyponatremia. Nevertheless, it's quite rare, and easily avoided if you simply drink sports drinks instead of water and drink according to your thirst rather than guzzling as much fluid as you can stomach. Preventing hyponatremia is not the most important reason to use a sports drink instead of water, but it is one more reason.

BENEFIT #2: MORE ENERGY

In long workouts, exhaustion can occur when the body's very limited stores of glycogen run low. The carbohydrate content of sports drinks provides a ready supply of glucose to the blood that the muscles can draw upon for energy. This allows the muscles to conserve glycogen when the sports drink is consumed at frequent intervals throughout the workout or race. The result is greater endurance.

Sports drinks also allow runners to work at a higher intensity level (i.e., go faster) in shorter workouts and races wherein glycogen depletion is not a concern. Exercise scientists are still puzzled as to why this is so. The probable explanation is that the brain is able to read the inflow of carbohydrate into the liver as a sign that it is "safe" to allow the muscles to work a little harder.

A pair of contrasting marathon performances by American record holder Deena Kastor presents an interesting case study providing evidence of the additive benefit of consuming carbohydrate along with fluid during running. The first of these two performances was at the 2004 US Olympic Trials Marathon held in St. Louis, Missouri. Kastor began as a heavy favorite to win, her best marathon time being 9 minutes faster than that of her nearest rival. Shockingly, however, Kastor "hit the wall" in the final miles, slowed down considerably, and lost her lead to Colleen de Reuck. Apparently worried that a regular sports drink would upset her stomach, Kastor chose to drink Pedialyte in this race, which contains water and electrolytes but no energy.

Fortunately, Kastor held on for second place and still made the Olympic team—and learned her lesson. In the Olympic Marathon staged 6 months later in Athens, she chose to use Cytomax, a sports drink containing 7 percent carbohydrate in addition to water and electrolytes. Despite stifling 100-degree heat, Kastor was able to run the second half of the race faster than the first, moving her way up from 28th place at the 5K mark to 3rd place and a bronze medal at the finish. Kastor's superior drink choice is almost certainly the primary reason she performed so much better in Athens than in St. Louis.

BENEFIT #3: LESS MUSCLE DAMAGE

While carbohydrate is the muscles' preferred energy source for moderate- to high-intensity exercise, during the latter portion of prolonged runs protein may supply as much as 15 percent of the muscles' energy needs. Most of the needed protein is taken from the muscles themselves, resulting in muscle tissue damage, soreness, and fatigue. In other words, in order to provide the energy they so desperately need, your muscles essentially eat themselves.

Because muscle protein breakdown is linked to muscle tissue damage, and also because protein is a less efficient energy source than carbohydrate, the body only begins to rely heavily on protein for energy as a last resort, after carbohydrate fuel supplies run low. As blood glucose and muscle and liver glycogen levels fall, a message is sent to the adrenal glands to release cortisol, the stress hormone that is responsible for breaking down proteins into their constituent amino acids, which are then converted into glucose in the liver.

Using a sports drink during running reduces muscle damage. The carbohydrate provided in the sports drink slows the rate of glucose and glycogen depletion and thereby reduces cortisol release, sparing muscle cells from "cannibalizing" themselves for energy.

Recent studies have shown that when athletes consume protein along with carbohydrate and fluid during exercise, muscle damage is substantially lower and endurance significantly greater than when carbohydrate and fluid are consumed without protein, as in a conventional sports drink. In fact, in one study, muscle damage was found to be 83 percent lower and endurance 29 percent greater with a carb-protein sports drink than with Gatorade, which contains no protein. The authors of this particular study apparently saw no connection between these two effects, but it seems quite likely that the reduction in muscle damage was itself a major reason the subjects given the carb-protein sports drink experienced delayed fatigue.

There are two theories about how the addition of protein to a sports drink might reduce exercise-related muscle damage. The protein in the sports drink may be used preferentially for energy during extended exercise, resulting in less breakdown of muscle protein. The supplemental protein may also raise amino acid levels in the blood.

Elevated levels of blood amino acids have been shown to reduce muscle protein breakdown.

BENEFIT #4: LOWER PERCEIVED EXERTION LEVEL

Perceived exertion is how running feels on a comfort–discomfort continuum. Scientists measure it with various qualitative and quantitative scales, but the bottom line is that the higher the level of perceived exertion, the more miserable you feel. Perceived exertion is important not only because feeling good feels good and feeling bad feels bad, but also because lower levels of subjective discomfort are associated with better running performance. In the past, high levels of perceived exertion were regarded as merely an effect of the true physiological causes of fatigue (glycogen depletion and so forth). Now they are believed to be as much a cause of fatigue as events in the blood, muscles, and elsewhere.

As you run, your brain receives feedback information from the muscles, blood, and other sources and uses this information to determine whether the body is in any way endangered. If it is, the brain then reduces muscle fiber recruitment, causing either a small or drastic reduction of pace. It also produces feelings of fatigue and discomfort that reduce the athlete's *willingness* to continue at the present pace. In *Lore of Running,* Tim Noakes, MD, puts it this way: "Fatigue is actually a central (brain) perception, in fact a sensation or emotion and not a direct physical event . . . [It] is merely the physical manifestation of a change in pacing strategy."

Without question, muscle glycogen and blood glucose levels are two of the primary factors that affect the "pacing strategy" that the brain selects. When either the muscle glycogen or the blood glucose level falls too low, the brain simply *causes* fatigue in order to make the runner slow to a pace that he or she can sustain (hopefully!) to the finish line. Drinking a carbohydrate sports drink during prolonged running is proven to reduce perceived exertion levels by keeping blood glucose levels higher. Drinking plain water during running has also been shown to reduce ratings of perceived exertion, but to a lesser extent. Carbohydrate and water work independently in this regard.

BENEFIT #5: LESS IMMUNE SYSTEM SUPPRESSION

Intense exercise suppresses the immune system for several hours. It does so by robbing the immune system of two of its principal fuels—glucose and the amino acid glutamine—and by stimulating cortisol release. One of the many effects of high cortisol levels is a reduction in immune system activity. This increases a runner's risk of contracting infections and it also hampers recovery, as the immune system plays an important role in healing muscle damage after exercise.

Conventional sports drinks reduce immune system suppression by providing glucose and by limiting cortisol release. Sports drinks containing glutamine (or whey protein, which is rich in glutamine) give the immune system an additional boost.

BENEFIT #6: FASTER RECOVERY

Sports drinks allow for faster post-exercise recovery by limiting dehydration and by reducing glycogen depletion, muscle damage, and immune suppression. As a result, it takes less time to rehydrate, replenish muscle energy stores, repair muscle damage, and regain full immune function.

BENEFIT #7: A BETTER WORKOUT TOMORROW

Believe it or not, using a sports drink during today's workout can actually enhance your performance in tomorrow's workout. It does this mainly by reducing muscle damage. Working out with residual muscle damage from previous training has been shown to reduce economy by 5 percent in runners, which is enough to severely compromise running performance.

DOES DEHYDRATION CAUSE HEAT ILLNESS?

Runners commonly assume that the reason they're supposed to drink to prevent dehydration while running is because dehydration causes heat stroke. This is a myth.

To begin with, doctors no longer use the term "heat stroke" in reference to an athlete collapsing during exercise in the heat. They now refer to "exertional heat illnesses" in the plural. Exertional heat stroke is the most severe form of exertional heat illness, wherein overheating causes significant damage to body tissues. Heat exhaustion is the diagnosis given when body temperature rises high enough to cause collapse but not high enough to cause significant tissue damage.

The word "exertional" gets at the true cause of these conditions, which is the accumulation of heat produced by the working muscles. The harder the muscles work, the more heat they produce. In hot weather (especially hot, humid weather), this excess body heat does not dissipate well and as a result it accumulates in the body. Exertional heat illnesses are most likely to occur during very intense exercise, when the muscles are producing the most heat. In these cases collapse occurs relatively quickly—long before dehydration has a chance to develop.

During prolonged exercise, body temperature rises as dehydration progresses. This is to be expected, since sweating is an important cooling mechanism that becomes less effective the longer it continues. However, it only goes so far. Even severely dehydrated runners seldom experience heat illness, and those who do are seldom more dehydrated than those who do not. There is evidence that some athletes are particularly susceptible to heat ill-

Conventional sports drinks reduce muscle damage by delaying glycogen depletion and thereby reducing the use of muscle proteins for fuel. As discussed earlier, sports drinks containing amino acids or protein in addition to carbohydrate reduce muscle damage even furness and therefore experience it at dehydration levels that aren't a problem for most.

This is not to suggest that dehydration is benign. The body temperature increase and the reduced blood flow that come with dehydration hamper running performance. And extreme dehydration can be fatal. However, athletic collapse is almost never caused by dehydration, which must exceed 15 percent to pose serious health risks. Very rarely do runners or other athletes reach levels of dehydration approaching even 10 percent. But dehydration levels of only 2 percent, which are very common during prolonged exercise, are sufficient to reduce endurance performance.

Drinking a sports drink during running lessens the performance-diminishing effects of dehydration and may slightly reduce the risk of heat illness in those who are susceptible. But the best way to prevent exertional heat illnesses is simply to avoid running in extremely hot weather, or at least to reduce the intensity and duration of your workouts in hotter weather.

It is possible to acclimatize to hot-weather running, and it's a good idea to do this before participating in long races that may take place in warm or hot weather. Heat acclimatization reduces sweat rate and the electrolyte concentration of sweat, allowing runners to slow the dehydration process somewhat when exercising in a hot environment. This process consists of gradually getting used to running in the heat over the course of 10 to 15 days. Start with a very short run at a very easy intensity on the first day and gradually increase the duration and intensity of running from day to day until you're able to run more or less normally in the heat.

ther. Given their superiority in reducing muscle damage, it's no surprise that carb-protein sports drinks have been shown to improve subsequent workout performance more than conventional sports drinks. In one study, athletes who used a carb-protein sports drink during a workout lasted 40 percent longer in a subsequent, exhaustive workout undertaken the following day than athletes who used a carb-only sports drink during the first workout.

CHOOSING THE RIGHT SPORTS DRINK

Many runners believe that all sports drinks are essentially the same. They are not. Differences in formulations that seem subtle on the labels may translate into highly disparate effects on your performance. Whereas one brand of sports drink might enhance your marathon performance by several percentage points as compared to water, another brand might cause you to cramp up, vomit, and fail to finish. There are several very good sports drinks on the market, but some so-called sports drinks don't even deserve the name. To make the best choice you need to know what to look—and look out—for on the labels. There are five items on this list: the types of carbohydrates, the concentration of carbohydrates, the amount of electrolytes, amino acids and protein, and useless extras.

TYPES OF CARBOHYDRATE

The best types of carbohydrate for fueling exercise are those that are easily broken down and absorbed by the stomach and intestine. These include sucrose (aka dextrose or table sugar), glucose, and maltodextrin, which is also called glucose polymers.

There are some carbohydrates, even "simple sugars" such as fructose, that are not as easily broken down and are more likely to cause gastrointestinal distress. Fructose actually slows down water and energy absorption, hampering energy and fluid delivery to your muscles. In addition, fructose has to be transported to the liver and converted to glucose before your muscles or brain can use it, making it a less efficient energy source than other carbohydrates that can bypass the liver. Galactose is another sugar that must pass through the liver first.

If a sports drink label lists fructose (or high fructose corn syrup) as the first or only carbohydrate, beware: It could lead to problems during prolonged exercise. A small amount of fructose in a sports drink won't cause problems as long as other, more easily absorbed sugars are also present. Fructose should be the second or third carbohydrate listed. Sucrose (dextrose), glucose, and/or maltodextrin (glucose polymers) should be listed above it.

A sports drink should also contain at least two, and ideally three types of carbohydrate. This is because different types of carbohydrate utilize distinct digestive pathways. If a sports drink contains only one type of carbohydrate, chances are it will overwhelm the pathway used to digest it, creating a backlog. But if a sports drink contains multiple types of carbohydrate, then multiple digestive pathways can process them simultaneously, so that glucose (always the end product) enters the bloodstream faster.

CARBOHYDRATE CONCENTRATION

Runners typically burn 100 to 200 grams of carbohydrate per hour at normal training intensities. But the average runner can absorb only 60 to 80 grams of ingested carbohydrate per hour. This means that even under the best of circumstances, runners cannot absorb enough carbohydrate to completely offset carbohydrate losses during running. What's more, even reaching the 60 to 80 grams per hour limit is far from automatic.

Two major factors affect how quickly carbohydrate is absorbed in fluid form. The first is stomach volume. The fuller your stomach is, the faster it empties. The second factor is the concentration of the fluid. Research has shown that carbohydrate is absorbed fastest when its concentration in a fluid is in the range of 6 to 8 percent (assuming normal drinking rates). Fluid itself is absorbed a little quicker when the carbohydrate concentration is somewhat less than 6 percent, but the actual rate of carbohydrate absorption is also a little lower because there's simply less carbohydrate provided.

There are some sports drinks with carbohydrate concentrations as low as 2 percent. Although they are absorbed quite quickly, they simply don't provide enough total carbohydrate and you should not use them unless you have a sensitive stomach and cannot tolerate sports drinks with the optimum 6 to 8 percent concentration.

In theory, a "sports drink" containing as much as 16 to 18 percent carbohydrate, although it is absorbed very slowly, could deliver carbohydrate at the maximum absorption rate of 60 to 80 grams per hour. However, it would require that a very large volume of fluid be maintained in the stomach, which is next to impossible during running. Consuming any sports drink containing more than about 8 percent carbohydrate at a realistic rate with a manageable stomach volume will result in a lower rate of nutrient delivery to the blood and muscles, and is more likely to result in GI distress.

ELECTROLYTES

Every sports drink should contain sodium, chloride, potassium, and magnesium. All four of these electrolytes are lost in sweat and your running performance will benefit from efforts to replace them. Only about half of the sports drinks on the market contain magnesium. Nearly all of them contain sodium and chloride (in the form of sodium chloride, or table salt), as well as potassium, but not always in adequate amounts. (Note that on most ingredient labels only the sodium content of sodium chloride is listed. Sodium and chloride exist in a 3:5 ratio in salt.)

The sweat of the average trained runner contains approximately 2,600 milligrams of sodium per liter, 1,100 milligrams of chloride per liter, 150 milligrams of potassium per liter, and 100 milligrams of magnesium per liter. In principle, a sports drink should contain these electrolytes in equal concentrations, but few existing sports drinks come anywhere close, in part because of palatability issues. My recommendation, therefore, is that you favor brands that contain the highest concentrations of electrolytes relative to the others.

Most sports drinks contain electrolytes in amounts that are adequate for normal training and racing. However, when you anticipate extreme sweat losses—for example in an ultramarathon—you will need to supplement your sports drink with salty foods such as pretzels (if possible) or salt tablets such as Lava Salts. In these circumstances, aim to take in 200 to 800 milligrams of sodium per hour.

AMINO ACIDS AND PROTEIN

Until recently, there was only one carbohydrate-protein sports drink on the market that I'm aware of: Accelerade. It contains 6 grams of whey protein per 12-ounce serving in addition to 7.75 percent carbohydrate. In independent studies (i.e., studies not funded by the manufacturer), this formula has been shown to drastically increase endurance and diminish muscle damage as compared to conventional sports drinks. One recent study found that it even hydrates better by boosting blood fluid retention.

There remains much to be learned about precisely how the addition of protein to a sports drink benefits athletes. New findings in this area may suggest further refinements in sports drink formulas. For example, it is probable that not every amino acid contained in whey protein carries a performance benefit. The sports drinks of the future will probably contain only select amino acids, not complete proteins. There is already research showing that the amino acids alanine and glutamine are especially beneficial during exercise. Cytomax contains both, and Revenge Sport contains glutamine, but in small amounts.

(continued on page 114)

A COMPARISON OF SEVERAL BRANDS OF SPORTS DRINKS

	Carbs % (main carb)	Electrolytes (per 12 oz)
Accelerade	6.5% (Sucrose)	190mg sodium 65mg potassium 128mg magnesium
All Sport	9% (High fructose corn syrup)	82mg sodium 75mg potassium
Cytomax	8% (High fructose corn syrup)	100mg sodium 110mg potassium
E3	7% (Sucrose)	250mg sodium 160mg potassium 150mg magnesium
Extran	5% (Fructose)	80mg sodium 66mg potassium
Gatorade	6% (Sucrose)	165mg sodium 45mg potassium
GU$_2$O	5.7%	180mg sodium 60mg potassium
Powerade	8% (High fructose corn syrup)	190mg sodium 65mg potassium
PowerBar	7% (Maltodextrin)	240mg sodium 15mg potassium 16mg magnesium
Revenge Sport	7% (Maltodextrin)	100mg sodium 110mg potassium 20mg magnesium
SoBe Sport	11% (Fructose)	105mg sodium 60mg potassium 12mg magnesium
Ultima Replenisher	2.5% (Maltodextrin)	78mg sodium 158mg potassium 20mg magnesium

Amino Acids/Protein	Other "Active" Ingredients
5 g whey protein concentrate	Vitamins C and E
—	Vitamins B_6, B_{12}, and C
Glutamine, alanine	Vitamin C
Glutamine, leucine, isoleucine, valine	Calcium and vitamin C
—	—
—	—
—	—
—	Vitamin B_6 and B_{12}
—	—
Glutamine	Vitamins C and E, ribose, and lactate buffers
—	Glucosamine, MSM, ribose, vitamins B_6 and B_{12}, and guarana
—	22 vitamins and minerals and CoQ10

E3 contains larger amounts of glutamine as well as the branched-chain amino acids leucine, isoleucine, and valine, which appear to be among the most beneficial amino acids to consume during exercise.

USELESS EXTRAS

One more thing to look out for is "marketing ingredients"—ingredients manufacturers boast on sports drink labels because they have a reputation for healthful effects, but which actually have no effect on performance and/or are included in amounts too small to have any physiological effect. Ribose, creatine, ginseng, CoQ10, and carnitine are some of the ingredients added to drinks to boost sales, not athletic performance.

For example, ribose is a sugar that became popular particularly among bodybuilders after preliminary research suggested that it enhances muscle recovery. Subsequent research showed that it does not, but ribose-containing supplements remain popular and it can still be found in a couple of sports drinks. Not only is ribose useless in any amount as a performance aid, but the drinks that contain it do so in such small amounts (0.05 grams in one case) that it would be useless anyway. Another drink contains about 2 milligrams of CoQ10, a coenzyme that has never been shown to improve athletic performance, and even if you take it for health reasons (it's an antioxidant), it needs to be consumed in amounts ranging from 30 to 100 milligrams.

The only ingredients besides water, carbohydrates, electrolytes, and protein/amino acids that are useful in a sports drink, based on current scientific knowledge, are the antioxidant vitamins C and E. These antioxidants are known to reduce exercise-related oxidative damage. However, it doesn't make any difference whether you get them during exercise or at other times.

WHAT ABOUT GELS?

Carbohydrate gels are essentially sports drinks without the water. Some gels (e.g., Clif Shot) contain electrolytes, while others (GU, for example) do not. In order to be absorbed as quickly as sports drinks are, gels must be consumed with water. And, of course, you need water anyway for hydration. If you use a gel that does not contain electrolytes, you need to get them from another source. That source should not be a sports drink because the combined carbohydrate concentration of gels and sports drinks is too great for optimal absorption. One option is to wash down your gels with an electrolyte-fortified water such as Pedialyte.

Gels (when taken with water) provide the same benefits as sports drinks and should be taken in the same circumstances. But you must choose one option or the other. The only sensible way to "combine" the two is by following gel consumption with water consumption for the next 20 to 30 minutes and then switching to a sports drink once the gel has been digested. So, when might you want to use gels instead of sports drinks?

- Some athletes simply prefer drinking water to sports drinks during exercise. If you are one of these athletes, you need to use gels.
- In some circumstances, gels are more convenient than sports drinks. For example, you can easily carry enough gel packets to fuel a 3-hour run and stop at water fountains for the water you need instead of being saddled with 2 or 3 pounds of sports drink in a hydration belt or fluid bladder.
- In races, if you are not a fan of the sports drink offered on the course, you can carry gel packets and just grab water cups from aid stations along the way.

■ In cool-weather workouts and races in which your sweat rate is relatively low but you're still burning lots of carbs, gels can be preferable to sports drinks. In such cases you will take the gels with somewhat less water than you would take in warmer weather. While this will slow the absorption rate slightly, it's better than having to urinate frequently, which is what will happen if you consume too much fluid while sweating lightly.

DRINKING GUIDELINES FOR WORKOUTS AND RACES

As already stated, I recommend that you use a sports drink during most if not all of your runs. Even in relatively short and easy runs wherein drinking will not affect your performance, it will still reduce muscle damage (especially if the drink contains protein) and accelerate recovery. You will also benefit from drinking in all races lasting an hour or more. Here are specific guidelines for drinking during workouts and races.

Use a fluid belt. The most convenient way to transport a sports drink on runs is to carry a squeeze bottle in a fluid belt. You can purchase these items at most running specialty shops. If you've never worn a fluid belt before or are not in the habit of doing so, you'll find it takes some getting used to; the constriction of the belt and the weight of the bottle against your lower spine are somewhat uncomfortable at first. In fact, the relative inconvenience of drinking on the run is the main reason that only a small fraction of competitive runners do so, whereas in sports such as cycling, in which transporting a bottle is more convenient, drinking throughout every workout is an almost universal practice. Nevertheless, I am certain that the benefits of drinking during runs outweigh the inconvenience.

When you're heading out for an easy run and you just aren't in the mood to be weighed down with even 8 or 12 ounces of fluid, at least make the effort to take a few swigs of your sports drink right before you start and immediately after you complete the run. If you are able to plan a route that passes a water fountain where you can wash down an energy gel somewhere in the middle, so much the better.

Drink during all high-intensity workouts. Drinking during the run itself should be 100 percent routine in all high-intensity workouts (e.g., intervals on the track) and in all runs of any intensity lasting an hour or longer. In these circumstances, drinking will enhance workout performance and thereby boost the training effect of the workout, in addition to reducing muscle damage, limiting immuno-suppression, and accelerating recovery. In long runs on roads or trails, you'll have to carry your drink. In high-intensity runs it's pro-hibitively cumbersome to carry fluid, and it's virtually impossible to drink while running at intensity levels above 10K race pace. I rec-ommend doing these workouts at a track or other venue where you can stash a squeeze bottle in a handy place and drink from it during jogging recoveries. Drinking between high-intensity intervals has been shown to enhance performance even in workouts lasting sig-nificantly less than an hour.

Drink small amounts frequently. Try to drink every 10 minutes or so throughout your workouts. Drinking frequently keeps your stomach volume higher, resulting in faster delivery of fluid and energy to the muscles. The precise amount you drink is not especially important. Research has shown that results are usually best when athletes drink *ad libitum*—that is, according to their thirst.

One exception is especially long workouts and races (2 hours plus) undertaken in warm or hot weather. In these circumstances, you should make an effort to drink at a rate that's as close as possible to your actual sweat rate. To determine your sweat rate, weigh yourself in the buff, on a scale with pounds and ounces, immediately before and immediately after a 60-minute run during which you do not drink. The number of ounces lost is your sweat rate per hour. Since your sweat rate is temperature-dependent, be sure to perform this test on a hot day if your objective is to figure out your target drinking rate for hot-weather running. Understand that it's very unlikely you'll actually be able to drink at 100 percent of your sweat rate while running; if you can comfortably replace two-thirds of losses you'll be fine.

Drinking during workouts also lets you practice before you try it during races. Individual runners vary significantly with respect to sweat rates and the amount of fluid and carbohydrate intake they can tolerate while running. Therefore, you need to experiment during training and determine exactly what works best for you so that you can duplicate it as closely as possible in races. Being able to drink comfortably while running is also a trainable skill, so practicing will not only help you determine how much you can tolerate but may also increase your tolerance.

Begin drinking before you start running. The first thing you need to do when it comes to training your gut for races is to start thinking about the contents of your stomach, or bolus. Because your stomach empties faster when it's fuller, it's a good idea to practice beginning your workouts with a larger bolus than you're used to having.

A sports drink is the ideal pre-run bolus builder because your bolus becomes running fuel as soon as you start running. The ideal time for bolus building is within minutes of beginning your run. Start by drinking a modest amount before running. Even a few ounces may feel uncomfortable at first, if you're used to running on an empty stomach, but keep doing it and you should adjust. When you do adjust, try drinking a little more before running, and continue in this way until you're confident you've found your personal limit.

Simulate race conditions. In at least some of your workouts, use the drink that will be offered at aid stations in the race you're training for. (It's usually named on the race Web site. If not, call the race management and ask.) If either your taste buds or your stomach does not react well to the race's sponsoring sports drink, or if the drink is poorly formulated (based on the guidelines given above), practice with it just a few times and use your preferred sports drink in your other workouts. Another option is to carry energy gels during the race and take only water from the fluid stations, in which case you'll need to practice using gels.

For drinking-practice purposes, carry or give yourself access to your sports drink during all of your long runs and race-pace workouts, because these are your most race-specific training sessions. It's especially important to practice drinking at race pace, because the faster you run, the harder drinking is mechanically and the less nutrition your stomach can tolerate. Again, begin by drinking only a small amount that you know you can handle. In subsequent workouts, gradually increase your intake until you reach the limit of your tolerance, keeping in mind that it may take your body a few tries to get comfortable with any given intake level. Increase your intake primarily by drinking more frequently rather than by drinking larger amounts at a time, because you'll maintain a larger bolus than you would if you drank the same amount but took larger swigs less frequently. Don't drink more often than once a mile, though, because you want to simulate the feeding schedule provided by race fluid stations.

Drinking is not beneficial in races lasting less than an hour. For legal reasons most race directors provide fluid stations in races even as short as 5K, and a great many runners take advantage of them, but it's silly. I can't help suspecting that the runners who guzzle greedily from paper cups in 5Ks are the same ones who never drink in training.

CHAPTER 6

PRE-RACE NUTRITION

When I was 11 years old my dad ran his first marathon. The night before the race our whole family ate spaghetti for dinner, at his request. Dad explained to my two brothers and me that he needed to "carbo-load" his muscles to help him go the distance. I can't recall exactly what carbo-loading meant to my preteen mind, but I know I got the general idea: that carbohydrates provide energy, that spaghetti provides carbohydrates, and that you need all the energy you can get to finish a marathon.

I know now that a single pasta dinner eaten the night before a marathon will not result in a significant carbo-loading effect and probably won't have any measurable effect on performance the next day, either. However, I've also learned that somewhat more sophisticated carbo-loading methods can be very effective. And, more generally, I've learned that the right approach to overall nutrition in the final days, hours, and minutes before a race can go a long way toward ensuring an optimal race performance, whereas a careless approach could sabotage your race in any number of ways.

Even if your everyday diet is flawless, you stand to benefit from tweaking your nutrition in a few key ways before a race, because a running race—especially a longer one—is not an everyday sort of challenge. In addition, it is important that you modify your training in ways that complement your pre-race nutrition strategy in order to render your body 100 percent race-ready when you toe the starting line.

Most of the pre-race nutrition strategies in this chapter apply only to longer races lasting 90 minutes or more. There is no benefit, for example, in carbo-loading prior to a race that will last fewer than 90 minutes. Other strategies, such as eating the perfect pre-race meal, are relevant to races of every distance.

CARBOHYDRATE LOADING

The practice of carbo-loading dates back to the late 1960s. The first carbo-loading protocol was developed by a Swedish physiologist named Gunvar Ahlborg after he discovered a positive relationship between the amount of glycogen in the body and endurance performance. Scientists and runners had already known for some time that eating a high-carbohydrate diet in the days preceding a long race enhances performance, but no one knew exactly why until Ahlborg's team zeroed in on the glycogen connection.

Subsequently, Ahlborg discovered that the muscles and liver are able to store above-normal amounts of glycogen when high levels of carbohydrate consumption are preceded by severe glycogen depletion. The most obvious way to deplete the muscles of glycogen is to eat extremely small amounts of carbohydrate. A second way is to engage in exhaustive exercise. The stress of severe glycogen depletion triggers an adaptive response by which the body reduces the amount of dietary carbohydrate that it converts to fat and stores, and increases the amount of carbohydrate that it stores in the liver and muscles as

THE AHLBORG CARBO-LOADING METHOD

1. Perform an exhaustive workout 1 week before a long race (90 minutes-plus).
2. Consume a very low-carb diet (10%) for the next 3 to 4 days while training lightly.
3. Consume a very high-carb diet (90%) the next 3 to 4 days while continuing to train lightly.

glycogen. Ahlborg referred to this phenomenon as glycogen super-compensation. Armed with this knowledge, he was able to create a more sophisticated carbo-loading protocol than the primitive existing method, which was, more or less, eating a big bowl of spaghetti.

Ahlborg came up with a 7-day carbo-loading plan in which an exhaustive bout of exercise was followed by 3 or 4 days of extremely low carbohydrate intake (10 percent of total calories) and then 3 or 4 days of extremely high carbohydrate intake (90 percent of total calories). Trained athletes who used this protocol in an experiment were able to nearly double their glycogen stores and exhibited significantly greater endurance in exercise lasting longer than 90 minutes.

After these results were published, serious endurance athletes across the globe began to use Ahlborg's carbo-loading plan prior to events anticipated to last 90 minutes or longer. (Meanwhile, less serious endurance athletes such as my father followed highly watered-down versions of it!) Although it worked admirably, it had its share of drawbacks. First of all, many athletes weren't keen on performing an exhaustive workout just a week before a big race, as the plan required. Second, maintaining a 10-percent carbohydrate diet for 3 or 4 days carried some nasty consequences, including lethargy, cravings, irritability, lack of concentration, and increased susceptibility to illness.

Many runners and other athletes found it just wasn't worth it. I myself never tried this carbo-loading protocol, but I know people who did and they were miserable during those depletion days.

Fortunately, later research showed that you can increase glycogen storage significantly without first depleting it. A newer carbo-loading protocol based on this research calls for athletes to eat a normal diet of 55- to 60-percent carbohydrate until 3 days before racing, and then switch to a 70-percent carbohydrate diet for the final 3 days, plus race morning. As for exercise, this tamer carbo-loading method suggests one final, longer workout (but not an exhaustive workout) done a week from race day followed by increasingly shorter workouts throughout race week. It's simple, it's nonexcruciating, and it works. Admittedly, some scientists and athletes still swear that the Ahlborg protocol is more effective, but if it is, the difference is slight and probably not worth the suffering and inherent risks.

Note that you should increase your carbohydrate intake not by increasing your total caloric intake, but rather by reducing fat and protein intake in an amount that equals or slightly exceeds the amount of carbohydrate you add. Combining less training with more total calories could result in last-minute weight gain that will only slow you down. Be aware, too, that for every gram of carbohydrate the body stores, it also stores 3 to 5 grams of water, which leads many athletes to feel bloated by the end of a 3-day loading period. The extra stored water is not a bad thing, though, considering that dehydration can be as big an issue as glycogen depletion in long races.

How do you know how much carbohydrate you're eating? It's easiest to count grams. In your normal diet, eating 6 to 7 grams of carbohydrate per kilogram of bodyweight (1 kg = 2.2 lb) will put you in the right percentage range. During the loading period, you should consume 10 to 11 grams of carbohydrate per kilogram of body weight. You can determine how many grams of carbohydrate various

THE NO-DEPLETION CARBO-LOADING METHOD

1. Perform a long workout (but not an exhaustive workout) 1 week before race day.
2. Eat normally (55 to 60% carbohydrate) until 3 days before a longer race.
3. Eat a high-carb diet (70%) the final 3 days before racing while training very lightly.

foods contain by reading labels and by consulting a book such as *The Complete Guide to Food Counts,* or by logging onto the USDA Nutrient Database at www.nal.usda.gov/fnic/foodcomp/search. As always, use high-quality carbohydrate sources such as whole grains rather than poor ones like cookies.

The newest and perhaps the best of all the carbo-loading strategies was devised in 2002 by scientists at the University of Western Australia. It combines depletion and loading and condenses them into a 1-day time frame. The creators of this innovative protocol recognized that a single, short workout performed at extremely high intensity creates a powerful demand for glycogen storage in both the slow-twitch and fast-twitch fibers of the muscles. They hypothesized that following such a workout with heavy carbohydrate intake could result in a high level of glycogen supercompensation without a lot of fuss. In an experiment, the researchers asked athletes to perform a short-duration, high-intensity workout consisting of 2½ minutes at 130 percent of VO_2max (about 1-mile race pace) followed by a 30-second sprint. During the next 24 hours, the athletes consumed 12 grams of carbohydrate per kilogram of lean body mass. This resulted in a 90 percent increase in muscle glycogen storage.

Runners have cause to be very pleased by these findings. Doing just a few minutes of high-intensity exercise the day before a competition

---

THE WESTERN AUSTRALIA CARBO-LOADING METHOD

1. During the pre-race week, eat normally while training lightly until the day before a longer race.

2. On the morning of the day before the race, perform a very brief, very high-intensity workout.

3. Consume 12 grams of carbs per pound of lean body mass (or 10 to 11 grams per pound of total body weight) over the next 24 hours.

---

will not sabotage tomorrow's performance, yet it will suffice to stimulate the desirable carbohydrate "sponging" effect that was sought in the original Ahlborg protocol. In fact, other research has shown that doing a little high-intensity running in the final days before a race is beneficial for reasons that have nothing to do with carbo-loading (more on this later). This allows the athlete to maintain a normal diet right up until the day before competition and then load in the final 24 hours.

Nevertheless, because it involves some very intense running, I don't recommend that you try this particular carbo-loading regimen for the first time before an important race. Test it initially before a shorter, less important race such as a 10K "tune-up" race that takes place several weeks before your marathon or other "peak" race. While carbo-loading won't actually affect your performance in a 10K, there's a slight chance that you won't recover well from even a small amount of high-intensity running done the day before any race. If you feel sore or flat in this test race, try doing the Western Australia carbo-loading regimen on the second to last day before your next race (e.g., on Friday if it's a Sunday race). As long as you rest and eat plenty of carbohydrate the following day, your muscles will still be glycogen loaded for your race.

Consuming 12 grams of carbohydrate per kilogram of lean body mass in a 24-hour period is easier said than done. For a 175-pound runner with 15 percent body fat this amounts to roughly 818 total grams of carbohydrate, or roughly the amount of carbohydrate you'll find in 18 servings of brown rice. The easiest way to get this much carbohydrate in a single day is to supplement normal-size meals comprising carbohydrate-rich foods with several servings of a carbohydrate-rich liquid supplement such as a meal replacement shake (e.g., Ensure, at 40 grams per can) or performance recovery drink (e.g., Endurox R[4] at 52 grams per 12-ounce serving). See page 128 for a sample of a 24-hour carbo-loading schedule.

Your pre-race dinner should be selected with special care. Once my wife made her special gumbo for my family the night before my brothers and I were to run a half-marathon together. The gumbo was delicious, but— please pardon my frankness—it set our bowels on fire the next morning. The moral of the story is that, besides choosing a meal that is rich in carbohydrate, you should also avoid foods that are likely to misbehave in one way or another once inside you. In particular, I would avoid spicy foods (gumbo, curry), greasy foods (fried seafood, french fries), and high-fiber foods (beans, onions).

A lot of runners have a ritual pre-race dinner. This is a good practice because it takes the worry and risk out of the situation. If your favorite pre-race dinner has always worked in the past, it will almost certainly work next time. Indeed, while there are dozens of menus that would probably work equally well on a strictly physical level, when you get down to within 16 hours of a big race and your nerves are raw, any little psychological boost is well worth getting. And the confidence that comes from eating a ritual pre-race dinner does provide a nice little boost for many runners.

When you're away from home for a race you have a little less control, of course. You can always rent a room with a kitchenette so you

SAMPLE 24-HOUR CARBO-LOADING SCHEDULE

This eating plan picks up immediately following the glycogen-depletion workout described on page 125, which should be performed first thing in the morning on the day before the race. It is designed to supply a hypothetical 175-pound runner with 15 percent body fat with approximately 818 grams of carbohydrate in the final 24 hours before racing.

Meal		Carbohydrates
Post-workout:	2 servings Endurox R[4]	104 g
Breakfast:	Oatmeal, orange juice	67 g
Midmorning snack:	Banana	
	Ensure	69 g
Lunch:	Peanut butter & jelly sandwich	
	Garden salad	
	Apple juice	82 g
Midafternoon snack:	Apple	
	Ensure	60 g
Predinner snack:	Endurox R[4]	52 g
Dinner:	Spaghetti w/ tomato sauce & roasted vegetables	
	Apple juice	110 g
Evening snack:	PowerBar	
	Ensure	85 g
Breakfast:	2 bananas	
	2 servings Endurox R[4]	162 g
Pre-race:	Energy gel	
	Water	27 g

can prepare your pre-race dinner just the way you like it, but in my view that's a little too uptight. I find it more relaxing to get away from the hotel and enjoy a good restaurant meal of the right basic type (I usually go for stir-fries) in the company of whomever I'm traveling with, trusting that the chef won't poison it. He never does.

TAPERING FOR OPTIMUM RACE FUELING

The Western Australia carbo-loading strategy works best if preceded by a proper taper—that is, by several days of reduced training whose purpose is to render your body rested, regenerated, and race-ready. In fact, several days of reduced training combined with your normal diet will substantially increase your glycogen storage level even before the final day's workout and carbohydrate binge. When you exercise vigorously almost every day, your body never gets a chance to fully replenish its glycogen stores before the next workout reduces them again. Only after 48 hours of very light training or complete rest are your glycogen levels fully compensated. Then the Western Australia carbo-loading regimen can be used to achieve glycogen supercompensation.

As with carbo-loading, various tapering strategies have been created and tested over the years. Believe it or not, in the early days of the modern sport of distance running few competitive runners even considered the idea that they should rest up prior to competing. The majority of them continued to train hard right up until race day itself. I don't believe these runners failed to notice that they tended to run best when well rested; rather, I suspect, they had an irrational fear of "losing fitness" as a result of not training hard even for a few days prior to racing. Almost every competitive runner has this irrational fear, and as a result even today many runners fail to taper properly despite the fact that its benefits are now scientifically proven.

Different tapering strategies are distinguished one from another by their duration, the size of the initial training volume reduction, how quickly training "decays" (i.e., the rate at which training volume is reduced from day to day) within the taper, and the intensity of workouts within the tapering period. Formal study of various tapering methods has revealed that the ideal length of a taper depends on the training volume preceding it and the length of the race that is to be run. The higher the training volume and the longer the race, the longer the taper should be. An elite marathoner who has been logging 120-mile weeks should taper for at least 2 weeks and possibly even 3 weeks. A 20-mile-a-week runner racing a 5K need not taper more than 2 or 3 days.

In addition, research has shown that the best results usually follow when there is a drastic initial drop in training volume (about 50 percent); when training decays steadily from day to day thereafter; and when a significant amount of high-intensity running (as a fraction of the total) is performed within the taper. In short, when your taper begins, slash your run length drastically, and then reduce it slowly and steadily each day thereafter. But continue to do a fair amount of high-intensity running (presuming you were doing a fair amount of high-intensity running prior to the taper).

This last property of the optimal taper—the retention of high-intensity training —is rather counterintuitive. You'd think that "resting up" for a race would require that you slash volume and intensity equally. However, it appears that doing almost as much high-intensity running within your taper as you did in the preceding weeks while reducing the amount of easy running results in a sudden enhancement of neuromotor efficiency. This is another reason to practice the Western Australia carbo-loading strategy described previously, as it calls for a very short high-intensity workout on the day before a race.

WHAT A MARATHON TAPER LOOKS LIKE

The following is an example of how the final 3 weeks of marathon training might look for a hypothetical runner maintaining a moderately high training volume and following a 2-week taper of the sort recommended in this chapter. Note that a final long run scheduled for 1 week prior to race day breaks the general pattern of a steady decay in volume. I always recommend doing a final longer run about a week before longer races (half-marathon and up) for maintenance of endurance adaptations.

Days Left Until Marathon	Training
20	Rest
19	10 miles (w/ 6-mile tempo)
18	8 miles easy
17	8 miles (w/ 3-mile intervals)
16	8 miles easy
15	8 miles easy + strides
14	24 miles
13	Rest
12	8 miles (w/ 5-mile tempo)
11	7 miles easy
10	6 miles (w/ 2.5-mile intervals)
9	6 miles easy
8	5 miles easy + strides
7	15 miles
6	Rest
5	5.5 miles (w/ 4-mile tempo)
4	3 miles easy + strides
3	4 miles (w/ 1.5-mile intervals)
2	Rest
1	2 miles (w/ 3-minute glycogen depletion interval)
—	Marathon

PRE-RACE HYDRATION

In addition to carbo-loading, many runners increase their fluid intake in the final days preceding a longer race to maximize their water stores and minimize dehydration during the race. Is this strategy really effective? It depends.

Studies have shown that pre-exercise hydration status does affect subsequent exercise performance. However, most of these studies compared endurance performance in a dehydrated state against performance in a state of normal hydration. The effect is much smaller when normally hydrated athletes are compared to over-hydrated athletes. In other words, if you drink enough generally, there is little to be gained from drinking more in the final day or two before a long race. And the effect of fluid loading disappears altogether when fluid is consumed consistently throughout the race itself.

What's more, simply drinking more fluid alone will not cause you to retain more water if you're already normally hydrated to begin with. You must also increase your intake of nutrients or compounds that enhance water retention. Otherwise, drinking more will only make you urinate more.

It so happens that carbohydrate is one of these nutrients. As I mentioned earlier, the muscles store 3 to 5 grams of water with each gram of glycogen. So carbo-loading and fluid loading go hand in hand. An important ramification of this fact is that optimal carbo-loading requires adequate water intake. This is a second reason to get much of the extra carbohydrate you need for carbo-loading in liquid form. The first reason, as I suggested earlier, is that it's simply easier to take in larger quantities of carbohydrate this way.

Another nutrient that increases water retention is sodium. Some ultrarunners and long-distance triathletes consciously increase their salt intake in the days preceding a race. However, they do so primarily to protect themselves against hyponatremia, not to increase water retention. This is just as well, because increasing your salt intake is unlikely to result in a meaningful amount of water retention unless your normal diet contains very little salt. The average American consumes 10 times the amount of salt needed for health, which means the average American is already retaining water due to sodium surpluses in the body. Additional salt intake is unlikely to yield much additional water retention because the kidneys are very good at getting rid of sodium faster when there's too much in the body.

A more effective water loading facilitator is glycerol. Glycerol is a natural compound that is similar in chemical structure to alcohol. It is present in the body in stored fat and in fluids and can also be purchased as a supplement. One effect of ingesting glycerol is an increase in blood plasma volume, which is potentially beneficial to athletes because it could slow the dehydration process during exercise.

Although the suggested dosage of glycerol depends on body size and varies between manufacturers, 1 gram per kilogram of body weight with an additional 1.5 liters of fluid taken 60 to 120 minutes before competition is standard. Studies on the effects of pre-exercise glycerol supplementation on athletic performance have produced mixed results. There is now general agreement that glycerol can increase endurance, but only in athletes who fail to drink enough before and during exercise. Since you should always hydrate adequately before and during exercise, glycerol supplementation is not necessary. Side effects including headaches and blurred vision are associated with excessive glycerol intake.

What's true for glycerol is true for water loading in general. Your focus should be on hydrating properly immediately before and throughout the race, as this is by far the most effective way to limit the performance-diminishing effects of dehydration. If you drink enough on race day, there will be little or no additional benefit in water loading before race day. And you will achieve some amount of water loading automatically as a side effect of carbo-loading.

A small downside of carbo-loading and the water retention that comes with it is weight gain. Competitive runners who carbo-load effectively typically show up on the starting line weighing 4 to 6 pounds more than they did just 1 or 2 days earlier. They can feel it, too: ponderous and somewhat bloated. There's no question that this added weight slows one down a little. But it's just as clear that the alternative is worse. Water and glycogen are performance-limiting resources in a longer race. Their extra availability will enhance performance more than their weight will harm it. And it will all be gone before you reach the finish line anyway.

THE PRE-RACE MEAL

Every meal is important, but no meal is more important than the last one you eat before a race. Choosing the wrong foods, eating too much or too little, or eating at the wrong time could completely ruin your race, or at least make your performance less than optimal. Eating the right pre-race meal at the right time will ensure that all your hard training doesn't go to waste.

The main purpose of the pre-race meal is to fill your liver with glycogen, especially if it precedes a morning race. Liver glycogen fuels your nervous system while you sleep, and as a result your liver is roughly 50-percent glycogen depleted when you wake up in the morning. Your muscles, inactive during the night, remain fully glycogen loaded from the previous day.

Timing is perhaps the most important consideration. The ideal time for a pre-race meal is about 4 hours before the race because it's early enough that you can digest and store a large amount of energy (i.e., a large number of calories), yet late enough that this energy won't be used up by race time. Most running races start early in the morning, and since sleep is also important, it's often impossible to eat a full breakfast 4 hours before the horn sounds. That's okay. It's usually possible to eat at least 2 hours out, and while you won't safely be able to eat as much this close to race time, you can still eat enough.

The appropriate size of your pre-race meal depends on three factors: the duration of your race, your size, and the timing of the meal. The longer the race you're competing in and the heavier you are, the larger your pre-race meal should be. The closer your pre-race meal falls to the race start, the smaller it must be. If you're able to eat 4 hours out, you can safely consume up to 1,000 calories. If you eat just 2 hours before the start, eat a smaller meal of 300 to 400 calories.

At least 80 percent of the calories you consume in your pre-race meal should come from carbohydrate. Keep your protein and especially your fat and fiber consumption low, because these nutrients will only take up space that would be better utilized by carbohydrate. Also avoid gas-producing foods such as onions.

The types of carbohydrate are not important. While some studies have shown a performance benefit associated with eating a low glycemic index (GI) meal rather than a high GI meal before exercise, these meals were eaten just 30 minutes before exercise, which is the worst possible time for a high GI meal, because the blood glucose level tends to decrease about 30 minutes after a high GI meal. (Recall that in a high GI meal, carbohydrates enter the bloodstream very quickly, whereas in a low GI meal, carbs enter the bloodstream at a lower rate.) In studies involving a more sensibly timed pre-exercise meal, the glycemic index of the meal has had no effect on performance. Choose foods and drinks that are not only easily digested, but also easily consumed, especially if you're prone to nervousness. Few athletes have their usual hearty appetite on race mornings, but the butterflies in their stomach usually permit consumption of soft, bland foods such as oatmeal and bananas. A liquid meal such as a breakfast shake is another good choice, as long as it's high in carbohydrate and low in protein, fat, and fiber. If you don't yet have a ritual pre-race meal, try various options and pay careful attention to the results. As with your pre-race dinner, once you've settled upon a pre-race breakfast that works well, stick with it.

Here are my choices for the five best foods to eat (or drink) before a race:

BAGEL

A bagel makes for an excellent pre-race breakfast food not only because it's rich in carbohydrate, bland, and easily digested, but also because it's something many runners eat for breakfast routinely, and therefore is familiar. Eat it dry or top it with something low in fat such as a light smearing of reduced fat cream cheese.

BANANA

Bananas are almost all carbohydrate. A large banana contains more than 30 grams of carbohydrate, just 1 gram of protein, and no fat whatsoever. Bananas are also extremely high in potassium (400 mg), which is lost in sweat during running. As mentioned above, their softness and light taste make them easy to consume even with pre-race nerves, and their natural "wrapper" makes them handy for eating on the road.

ENERGY BAR

Energy bars such as PowerBar and Clif Bar are made to be eaten before exercise. Most are very high in carbohydrate and low in fiber, fat, and protein. The better bars also contain useful amounts of sodium, potassium, and the antioxidant vitamins C and E. A cappuccino flavored PowerBar, for example, contains 45 grams of carbohydrate,

110 milligrams each of sodium and potassium, 35 percent of the recommended daily allowance of magnesium, and 100 percent of the RDA of vitamins C and E.

There's a huge variety of energy bars on the market and some are better than others. Choose one that's close to the PowerBar formula I just outlined. Avoid the high-protein, low-carb bars that have become popular in recent years. The advantage of the wide selection of bars on the market is that it's easy to find one you like and can eat without unpleasantness before a race. Pay attention to texture, too. Some bars are very chewy, and for some runners (myself included) eating chewy foods tends to exacerbate the stomach churning that's associated with pre-race nervousness.

MEAL REPLACEMENT SHAKE

I drink one or two meal replacement shakes before almost every race. Brands such as Boost and Ensure have nearly the perfect nutrition profile, plus they take care of energy and hydration needs simultaneously, they're superconvenient, and nothing is easier to consume before a race, even if you're extremely anxious. And they taste good. Ensure, for example, delivers a whopping 250 calories of energy in a little 8-ounce can, including 40 grams of carbohydrate. The one downside to these beverages providing so much nutrition in so little volume is that they are not as filling as solid foods and can actually leave you feeling a little hungry in the middle of a marathon if you rely on them solely.

In the same general category as meal replacement shakes, for the purpose of pre-race fueling, are performance recovery drinks including Endurox R[4] and Ultragen, which are normally used immediately after exercise. They are sold as powders that you mix with water. Because these drinks are slightly more dilute than meal replacement drinks, they do an even better job of hydrating and fueling simultaneously.

OATMEAL

Like bananas, oatmeal is almost pure carbohydrate and is soft and light in taste. It is also the most filling among the five best pre-race foods, which is good for those who want to feel something substantial in their belly before they head out to burn a few thousand calories. Some runners also prefer to eat a real breakfast food for breakfast, and oatmeal is certainly that.

Oatmeal requires preparation that can be more challenging on the road than at home. If your hotel room has a microwave oven, you're all set as long as you've brought some kind of bowl with you. If there's no microwave oven, you can use the coffee maker to heat water.

THE FINAL TOUCHES

Between the time you eat your pre-race meal and roughly 1 hour before the race start, sip at regular intervals from a bottle of sports drink or electrolyte-fortified water (e.g., Propel). Don't go overboard; just drink enough to keep your urine clear in color. Don't drink between 60 minutes and 10 minutes prior to the race. This is the time for the fluid you have consumed to go where it's needed and for any excess to be shunted to your bladder so you can get rid of it. If you make the mistake of continuing to drink during this interval you may find yourself needing to urinate during the race, which is no fun. Another advantage of drinking something containing electrolytes at this time is that it limits the excretion of water through the kidneys, so less water winds up being lost to your bladder.

Between 60 and 30 minutes before the horn sounds you may wish to take one or two caffeine pills. Caffeine is the common name for the drug trimethylxanthine, a natural alkaloid compound that functions in the body mainly as a mild nervous system stimulant. It has been shown to enhance performance in sprints, in all-out efforts lasting 4 to 5 minutes, and in prolonged endurance exercise.

It appears caffeine enhances performance in shorter events by increasing muscle recruitment. In longer events it delays fatigue by reducing the athlete's perception of effort. It increases the concentration of hormonelike substances in the brain called beta-endorphins during exercise. The endorphins affect mood state, reduce perception of pain, and create a sense of well-being.

Caffeine has also been found to delay fatigue during exercise by blocking adenosine receptors. Adenosine is produced during exercise and inhibits the release of the brain neurotransmitter dopamine. Decreases in dopamine, along with increases in serotonin, another brain neurotransmitter, have been linked to central nervous system fatigue during exercise.

The performance-enhancing effects of caffeine decrease with habituation to caffeine intake, so it's best to eliminate caffeine consumption for several days before racing. Also, pure caffeine pills are more effective than other caffeine sources such as coffee. Some energy gels contain caffeine, but not in amounts sufficient to have much of an effect on their own. Recommended intake is 5 to 6 milligrams per kilogram of body weight 60 to 30 minutes before racing.

About 10 minutes before the start of your race, it's time to create your bolus. In the previous chapter, I defined a bolus as the contents of your stomach. Creating a relatively large bolus before running (especially a race) is desirable because the fuller your stomach is, the faster it empties, and the faster your stomach empties, the faster it delivers fluid and energy to your blood and muscles while you run. It's important to wait until just a few minutes before the race start to create your bolus, because cutting it this close ensures that most of what you drink will still be in your stomach (rather than your bladder) when you begin to run. Drink several swigs of sports drink or swallow a gel packet with several swigs of water or electrolyte solution. From practicing bolus-building in training you should know the maximum amount of fluid you can take in at this time without experiencing gastrointestinal troubles when you start running, and that's precisely how much you should drink.

Note that a small percentage of runners do not respond well to taking in carbohydrate within an hour before running. They experience a significant drop in blood glucose levels and consequently feel fatigued almost from the very first stride. The race-day nutrition plan I've just outlined should work well even for these runners, as the only carbohydrate consumed within the hour before running is consumed almost immediately before running and therefore functions the same way as carbs taken in during running.

In recent years, since the advent of the low-carb craze, I've encountered increasing numbers of runners who avoid consuming carbohydrate before racing not because they don't respond well to it but rather because they have been taught to fear an "insulin spike" and subsequent "blood sugar crash." This is a misplaced fear. Exertion prevents any such thing from occurring except in the small minority of runners just described. Insulin and blood glucose levels are tightly regulated during exercise. It's best to think of it this way: Any carbohydrate that's in your body when you start running is carbohydrate that can be used to fuel your running, so the more the better.

CHAPTER 7

RECOVERY NUTRITION

During the original running boom of the 1970s, a macho, no-pain-no-gain mentality pervaded the elite ranks of the sport. The top runners did not just try to outrun one another in races; they also tried to out train one another between races. They gave no credence to the notion of overtraining. Rather, they believed that the "right" amount of training equaled the most they could possibly train without breaking down and failing to make it to the starting line. Only a few runners—who were scoffed at by everyone else—believed that training too much might actually cause performance to diminish even in the absence of major injuries. Runners who admitted to valuing recovery were considered wimps.

Looking back, it's no surprise that this era was littered with the carnage of supremely talented runners who destroyed their bodies in the prime of life and therefore never realized their full athletic potential. Perhaps the most salient cautionary tale is that of Alberto Salazar. Born in Cuba and raised in the United States, Salazar was, in his brief heyday (1979–1983), probably the most gifted distance runner who had ever lived to that time. He won the New York City Marathon three times as well as the 1982 Boston Marathon, setting an American record and becoming the first runner ever to record two sub-2:09 marathons.

Talent alone did not elevate Salazar to this level of performance. He trained with maniacal zealotry, packing week after week with murderous workouts, seldom indulging in easy runs, scarcely doing anything resembling recovery, and never taking time off during the off-season. But while this over-the-top approach did take him to the top of the marathoning world in the short term, it was not sustainable for the long term. Salazar's career came completely unraveled when he was only 26 years old. He finished a humiliating fifteenth in the 1984 US Olympic Trials Marathon, and it only got worse.

Salazar developed a condition that is now known as overtraining syndrome. It is caused by a pattern of too much training and too little rest that is sustained over a long period of time and can be exacerbated by competitive pressures, poor diet, poor sleep, illness, and other factors. Often the first sign is an unexpected stagnation in performance, which is usually followed by a clear performance downturn. Among the many other signs and symptoms that also follow are muscle soreness, chronic fatigue, depression, irritability, apathy, weight loss, susceptibility to infection, and gastrointestinal disturbances—most of which Salazar did indeed experience. In fact, he became so sick that he failed to recover until many years after he had quit competitive running.

Overtraining syndrome is what's called a maladaptation (or, negative adaptation) to exercise stimulus. The part of the body that is at the root of this maladaptation is the endocrine system, and in particular a set of three glands—the hypothalamus, the pituitary, and the adrenals—known collectively as the HPA axis. The HPA axis produces and regulates the hormones that respond to stressors of all kinds, including the stress of training. When a manageable training load is combined with adequate rest, the HPA axis becomes stronger. When a runner persistently overtrains, the HPA axis essentially becomes exhausted, resulting in chronically low levels of vital hormones such as adrenaline and cortisol. Because these hormones play roles in virtually every part of the body, a long list of signs and symptoms may result.

Overtraining syndrome is fairly rare and is seen almost exclusively in elite athletes who are capable of maintaining prodigious training loads for months on end without suffering a disabling injury. I mention it here as an extreme example of the consequences of inadequate recovery, which is bad in any amount. While it takes a massive recovery deficit to trigger overtraining syndrome, even a small one could take the edge off your race performances or cause an avoidable injury.

What does nutrition have to do with this? You'll soon see.

THE INGREDIENTS OF RECOVERY

Individual workouts stress your body by depleting energy supplies, disrupting muscle tissue, suppressing the immune system, and affecting the function of other body systems. This type of stress is often referred to as a training stimulus. After the workout is completed, your body initiates various physiological processes designed to restore homeostasis, which is a fancy way of saying your body tries to return to the state it was in before the workout. These processes include replenishing muscle energy stores, building new muscle proteins, restoring resting hormonal patterns, and a variety of other responses. Collectively, the various processes that lead back to homeostasis constitute recovery.

There is a very close relationship between acute recovery (the body's short-term response to a single training stimulus) and adaptation (the body's longer-term response to repetitive training stimuli). You can think of recovery as a series of short trips that add up to the lengthy voyage of adaptation, or fitness gains.

Consider the example of muscle glycogen storage. An individual workout sharply reduces muscle glycogen stores. After the workout, your body automatically replenishes these stores. But the stress of exercise-induced glycogen depletion also affects the genes that are responsible for determining the maximum limit of glycogen storage. In response to exercise, these genes are "upregulated" to produce more of the key proteins involved in glycogen storage. As a result, consistent exercise quickly leads to an increase in the capacity of the muscles to store glycogen, which allows you to run farther before becoming fatigued. This is just one among dozens of ways in which a series of immediate post-workout recoveries becomes an important fitness adaptation over time.

Optimal recovery is the amount of recovery required to perform well in your next workout (assuming a sensible training schedule). It is not necessary or even possible to achieve a positive, adaptive response to each workout before you begin your next one. In fact, it's not always necessary even to achieve homeostasis (for example 100-percent glycogen replenishment) between workouts. What matters is that, on balance, key aspects of your recovery are able to reach a point between workouts that allows you to train progressively over the course of many weeks.

Post-exercise recovery has three ingredients: time, rest, and nutrition. Some aspects of recovery happen faster than others. For example, under normal circumstances post-workout muscle inflammation abates faster than muscle glycogen is fully restored. But no aspect of recovery happens instantaneously, so if you don't allow enough time between workouts, you won't recover adequately. In addition, all recovery processes require inactivity or relatively low activity levels to proceed swiftly and without interruption. Since it is the intense activity of running that creates the need for recovery, doing some other type of intense activity between runs will not facilitate your recovery. This may seem obvious, but I have known a few runners who've behaved as though they didn't know it.

Finally, as I mentioned in Chapter 1, virtually all recovery processes unfold through the medium of nutrition. You cannot replenish glycogen stores, for example, without consuming carbohydrate between workouts. The right approach to recovery nutrition can make a huge difference in how quickly and thoroughly you recover from each workout.

RECOVERY NUTRITION

There are five specific effects of exercise on the body that immediate post-exercise recovery nutrition can address. Based on those effects, the five goals of recovery nutrition are as follows:

- Rehydration
- Replenishing muscle glycogen
- Reducing secondary muscle damage and preventing illness
- Rebuilding muscle proteins
- Replenishing muscle fat stores

It is important that you begin the recovery nutrition process as soon as possible after completing each workout (and race), for a few reasons. Most obviously, the above-mentioned recovery processes depend on particular nutrients, so they can't even begin until you eat or drink. So the sooner you eat and drink, the faster and more thoroughly you will recover and the sooner you will be ready to perform well in a subsequent workout. Also, some of these processes will happen more rapidly during the first hour after exercise than at any later time—again, provided you get the proper nutrients. The balance of certain key hormones during the first hour or so after exercise—a period often called the recovery window—renders your body especially ready to make the best use of the nutrients it needs for recovery. Finally, exercise-related muscle damage can actually continue for some time after you finish exercising unless you quickly consume carbohydrate and protein to lower cortisol levels and initiate muscle protein rebuilding. For these reasons, consider your runs incomplete until you've begun to consume your recovery nutrition.

REHYDRATION

Except in cases when you run slowly in cool or cold weather and guzzle fluids the whole way, you are at least mildly dehydrated after every run. Exactly how much fluid you lose during any given run depends on several factors. The factors that are positively correlated with sweat loss are run duration and intensity, body mass, air temperature, humidity, altitude (which affects water loss through breathing, not sweating), heat acclimatization (which is relevant only in hot weather), and fitness level (the higher your VO_2 max, the higher your sweat rate). Genetic factors also influence sweat rate. In temperate weather, typical sweat loss rates in runners fall in the range of 800 to 1,200 milliliters per hour, but in higher temperatures and at higher intensities the rate of sweat loss can climb to well in excess of 2 liters per hour.

Drinking a sports drink throughout your runs can partially replace sweat losses and limit your level of dehydration after the run. You can estimate the amount of sweat lost during a run by weighing yourself in the buff on a scale (accurate to the ounce) immediately before and immediately after the run. To return to full hydration status within the next several hours you need to consume 1.5 ounces of fluid for each ounce of weight you lost during the run. The reason you need to drink more fluid than you lost is that you will continue to lose fluid through urination, breathing, and perspiration through the remainder of the day.

As with hydration during exercise, drinking plain water is not adequate for rehydration after exercise. Plain water does not exist anywhere in your body. All body fluids, including sweat, are full of electrolytes, so you have to replace your lost electrolytes along with water. And again, plain water is not absorbed by the body as well as electrolyte solutions. Therefore, your postrun drink probably should be a sports drink, performance recovery drink, or fitness water containing relatively large amounts of sodium chloride, potassium, and magnesium. If you do drink plain water, take it with foods containing adequate amounts of these minerals.

REPLENISHING MUSCLE GLYCOGEN

Your muscles use carbohydrate (glycogen and glucose) at a rate of 2 to 6 grams per minute during running. As with sweat rate, the rate of carbohydrate use depends on several factors, including the run intensity, air temperature, your fitness level, and genetic factors. The duration of your run affects the total amount of carbohydrate used. Your leg muscles always suffer the greatest carbohydrate (specifically glycogen) losses because they have the greatest initial supply and it is used preferentially during running.

Since the rate of carbohydrate use is affected by many of the same factors as the rate of sweat loss, you can actually use sweat loss to get a rough estimate of the amount of carbohydrate you lost during a run. For every 4.5 ounces of sweat you lose, your muscles burn roughly 100 total calories. In a typical workout, about 80 percent of these calories come from carbohydrate. Suppose your measured weight (sweat) loss after a run is 18 ounces. Divide 18 by 4.5 and multiply the product (4) by 100 to determine the rough total number of calories burned: 400. Now multiply 400 by 0.80 to figure out the approximate number of carbohydrate calories: 320. Since there are approximately 4 calories in each gram of carbohydrate, you can also calculate that you lost in the neighborhood of 80 grams of carbohydrate during the run.

These calculations work only if you drank nothing during the run. If you did drink, you need to add the volume of water consumed to the amount of weight you lost during the run and use this total as the basis for calculating the amount of carbohydrate burned. If you drank water, you can leave it there. If you drank a sports drink or anything else containing carbohydrate, there's one more step. Once you've figured out how many grams of carbohydrate you burned during the run, you need to subtract from this number the amount of carbohydrate you consumed during the run. This will yield your net carbohydrate deficit.

Let's look at an example. Suppose you complete a long run weighing 24 ounces (1.5 pounds) less than you did when you started. During the run, you drank 12 ounces of Gatorade. Add the 12 ounces of Gatorade to the 24 ounces of weight lost to calculate the actual amount of sweat loss: 36 ounces. Divide 36 ounces by 4.5 and multiply by 100 to determine the number of calories burned: 800. Multiply 800 by 0.80 to determine the number of carbohydrate calories burned: 640. Divide 640 by 4 to convert the result to grams of carbohydrate: 160. Now, according to its label, Gatorade contains 21 grams of carbohydrate per serving, and you consumed exactly 3 servings, or 63 grams of carbohydrate. Finally, subtract 63 grams from 160 grams to determine your carbohydrate deficit after the run: 97 grams.

To feel good and perform well in your next run, you need to get your glycogen levels back to normal beforehand. This is usually not difficult if you consume plenty of carbohydrate on a daily basis.

Incidentally, if you were a frog, you wouldn't have to worry so much. Frogs and some other animals can replenish muscle glycogen even while fasting by converting lactate into glycogen. But as humans we have no option but to chow down. In a study, athletes in heavy training who ate a low-carbohydrate diet (5g/kg/day, or 2.25g/lb/day) failed to fully replenish their muscle glycogen stores between workouts, while those who ate double that amount of carbohydrate replenished it easily. If you train moderately hard, 4 grams of carbohydrate per pound of body weight per day is a good mark to shoot for.

Achieving full glycogen replenishment between workouts is easier if you consume carbohydrate within the first hour after working out. Exercise-induced muscle glycogen depletion turns the muscle fibers into veritable carbohydrate sponges, in part by making them highly insulin sensitive but also through an insulin-independent mechanism that is not yet well understood. But these effects are transient. Consequently, carbohydrate consumed immediately after exercise may result in twice the amount of glycogen synthesis as the same amount of carbohydrate consumed 3 hours later. You can maintain an elevated rate of glycogen synthesis for 4 to 5 hours by consuming a carbohydrate snack every half-hour throughout this time period. The highest rate of glycogen synthesis is achieved when carbohydrate is consumed with a modest amount of protein, because amino acids stimulate additional insulin release, resulting in faster transport of glucose and amino acids to the muscles.

If you work out twice a day some days (called "doubling"), immediate post-workout carbohydrate intake is even more important. When you double, fully replenishing your muscle glycogen stores in the 4 to 8 hours between workouts is practically impossible, so it's crucial that you replenish them as fully as you can. Studies have shown that athletes perform much better in an afternoon workout when they take in adequate carbohydrate immediately after a morning workout. To ensure the highest level of performance in your afternoon workout, consume your immediate post-workout carbs with a little protein and have a few small carbohydrate snacks at 30- to 60-minute intervals thereafter.

How much carbohydrate do you need after running? Shoot for an amount equal to between 50 percent and 100 percent of your total carbohydrate deficit within the first hour after completing each run. After a shorter run it's usually fairly easy to make up the full deficit quickly. After a longer workout such as that in the preceding example, it's a little more challenging (97 grams is a lot of carbohydrate!). In these instances, aim for at least 50 percent of the deficit.

REDUCING SECONDARY MUSCLE DAMAGE AND PREVENTING ILLNESS

The short-term effect of strenuous exercise on the immune system is complex, as is the immune system itself. On the one hand, strenuous exercise drains the immune system of two of its principal fuels: glucose and the amino acid glutamine, which is metabolized at a higher rate than any other amino acid during exercise. An especially long or hard run also results in high levels of circulating cortisol, which further suppresses the immune system. The consequence of these effects is a heightened susceptibility to infections during the hours following a hard run.

On the other hand, exercise-induced muscle damage triggers an inflammation response—itself a type of immune response—that can easily get out of hand and cause a significant amount of additional muscle damage. After exercise, immune cells travel to the muscles and begin the repair process by removing cellular debris. As they work, these immune cells release toxins and free radicals that cause further damage to parts of the muscle cell. This phenomenon is referred to as secondary muscle damage because it occurs after the workout is completed, and it can continue for as long as 3 days afterward (in extreme cases). This is why muscle damage (and muscle soreness) usually hit a peak 1 to 3 days after hard exercise rather than immediately afterward.

Limiting secondary muscle damage and preventing illness after exercise go hand in hand because both objectives require immune system modulation. In order to limit muscle damage, you need to take in nutrients that limit inflammation and free radical damage. Antioxidant vitamins, especially vitamins C and E, tend to reduce secondary muscle damage caused by free radicals after exercise. It's not especially important to consume these vitamins within the recovery window. It's enough that your everyday diet be rich in vitamins C and E, perhaps with the help of vitamin supplements. In fact, if you consume enough vitamin C and vitamin E on a daily basis you will suffer significantly less primary muscle damage during exercise, in addition to less secondary muscle damage after exercise. Foods rich in vitamin C include citrus fruits and juices, broccoli, and mustard greens. Foods rich in vitamin E include green leafy vegetables, whole grains, nuts and seeds, and eggs.

Omega-3 fatty acids are a powerful anti-inflammatory nutrient. They are nutrient precursors of anti-inflammatory prostaglandins that help keep the inflammatory response to primary muscle damage from getting out of control. As with vitamins C and E, there is no rush to get omega-3 fatty acids into your body within the recovery window. It takes time for your body to manufacture prostaglandins from omega-3 fatty acids, so it's enough just to maintain an everyday diet that's rich in these nutrients. Good sources of omega-3 fatty acids include wild salmon, halibut, soy, flaxseeds, and grass-fed organic beef.

In order to lower your susceptibility to infection after exercise, you need to consume carbohydrate and glutamine during and after workouts and races. The use of a carbohydrate sports drink during and after running has been shown to drastically reduce immunosuppression and lower infection rates in runners. Taking in glutamine (especially after running) is proven to do the same.

REBUILDING MUSCLE PROTEINS

Cortisol damages muscle cells during exercise by dismantling muscle proteins so that the body can use the amino acids they consist of for energy. Cortisol levels tend to remain high for some time following exercise; this is another reason muscle damage often continues long after a run is completed. Ironically, one of cortisol's main jobs after exercise is to limit inflammation, which, as just noted, itself causes further muscle damage after exercise.

To limit post-exercise muscle damage and accelerate the repair process you need both protein and carbohydrate. Protein and amino acids, the main structural components of muscle tissue, are the most important nutrients for rebuilding. Numerous studies have shown that protein synthesis in the muscles occurs more rapidly when protein and/or amino acids are consumed immediately after exercise. However, the muscles can use only a limited amount of amino acids during the acute recovery period, something that strength athletes who guzzle protein shakes after exercise would do well to learn.

The hormonal environment in the body can slow down protein synthesis, and that's where carbohydrate can make a major difference. Carbohydrate stimulates insulin production, which reduces muscle protein breakdown and accelerates muscle protein synthesis after exercise. When blood insulin levels rise, cortisol levels fall. At the same time, insulin also delivers both glucose and amino acids to the muscles and even increases blood flow to the muscles. In fact, the fastest rates of post-exercise muscle protein synthesis are achieved when a modest amount of protein or amino acids is consumed with a fairly large amount of high-glycemic carbohydrates (approximately 3 to 6 grams of carbohydrate per gram of protein). Many foods and meals fall within this range, including breakfast cereal with low-fat milk, a turkey sandwich, and sushi.

Interestingly, just as carbohydrate facilitates muscle repair, protein facilitates muscle glycogen replenishment after exercise. This is because muscle tissue damage is one of the major limiters of post-exercise muscle glycogen replenishment. When muscle cells are damaged, they are not able to synthesize glycogen normally. By facilitating muscle repair, protein and amino acids consumed after exercise also promote glycogen replenishment.

REPLENISHING MUSCLE FAT STORES

It is often remarked that the body contains a virtually unlimited supply of fat fuel, whereas the supply of carbohydrate fuel is quite limited. Consequently, although we know runners burn a lot of fat during running, they are seldom advised to worry about "replenishing" fat stores after exercise.

However, not all fat is equally accessible as running fuel. The portion of our total body fat stored in our muscles—called intramuscular triglycerides—is most accessible as muscle fuel and therefore the body uses it preferentially during running. But these stores are indeed quite limited. Fat stored in the leg muscles decreases by about two-thirds during an exhaustive run. That's about the same level of depletion that muscle glycogen stores reach at the end of an exhaustive run. So replenishing intramuscular triglycerides after running is actually as important as replenishing muscle glycogen.

Just as the key to full glycogen replenishment between workouts is adequate carbohydrate intake, the key to full replenishment of intramuscular triglycerides between workouts is adequate fat consumption. In one study, cyclists who ate a 24 percent fat diet failed to fully replenish their muscle fat stores within 48 hours after a 3-hour workout, while cyclists who ate a 39 percent fat diet did regain pre-workout levels of muscle fat within this time frame. These results should not necessarily be taken to mean that *you* should maintain a diet of 39 percent fat, but they do suggest that runners probably need a higher fat diet than sedentary persons need. (Remember that runners who maintain very low-fat diets are more likely to get injured than those who eat more fat.)

There has been little research into the effects of the timing of post-workout fat intake. Because fats have a strong tendency to slow gastric emptying—with the result that it takes longer for the digestive process to deliver fluid, carbohydrate, and protein to your blood and muscles—I recommend that you eat little or no fat during the first hour after training. But be sure to get plenty of fat from good sources (nuts, fish, olive oil) at other times.

ENGINEERED RECOVERY DRINKS VERSUS NATURAL RECOVERY FOODS

In the past several years, special post-workout recovery drinks (most of them sold in powdered form) have become quite popular among runners and other athletes. The makers of these drinks want us to believe that they are a better choice for recovery nutrition than meals consisting of everyday foods such as sandwiches and fruit. Is this true?

In the absence of any good research exploring this question, I believe that a runner who consistently eats the right foods (and drinks enough fluid) within the recovery window will be no worse off than a runner who drinks a good recovery drink. Nevertheless, I use recovery drinks, because they do have some practical advantages over regular foods after exercise.

Drinks are easier to consume when you're not hungry. Most runners have little appetite during the first hour after a run—especially after

WHAT MAKES A GOOD RECOVERY MEAL?

To get your recovery nutrition primarily from foods, choose foods (and beverages) that meet your specific recovery nutrition needs, and eat them within the recovery window (i.e., the first hour after completing your workout). The following meals offer enough protein and carbohydrate for optimal recovery.

Recovery Breakfast

Toast with peanut butter

Large glass of orange juice

Water

Recovery Lunch

Turkey sandwich with lettuce and mustard on whole grain bread

Banana

Large glass of apple juice

Water

Recovery Dinner

Spaghetti with tomato sauce and meatballs (lean beef or turkey)

Garden salad with olive oil and vinegar dressing

Glass of water

a hard run. This happens in part because running causes the hypothalamus gland—the brain's hunger center—to release some of the same neurotransmitters that tell you you're full after eating a meal. Hunger is also suppressed when there are high levels of amino acids and fatty acids in the blood, as is the case after exercise due to the mobilization of these nutrients to provide energy during running. High-intensity running increases plasma amino acid levels more than low- to moderate-intensity running, which may explain why high-intensity running suppresses hunger more.

At the same time, the dehydration that results from sweating during

COMPARISONS OF POST-WORKOUT RECOVERY DRINKS

Product	Calories	Carbs	Protein	Fat	Key Amino Acids
Countdown	244	42 g (Dextrose)	14 g (Whey protein concentrate)	1.5 g	2 g BCAA 1 g glutamine
Cytomax Recovery	348	18 g (Amylopectin)	26 g (Casein)	18 g	5 g BCAA 3.75 g glutamine
Endurox R⁴	270	52 g (Dextrose)	13 g (Whey protein concentrate)	1.5 g	2.7 g BCAA 420 mg glutamine
GNC Pro Performance Powerload	162	32 g (Maltodextrin)	6 g (Whey protien concentrate)	1 g	361 g BCAA 250 mg glutamine
PowerBar Performance Recovery	135	30 g (Maltodextrin)	4.5 g (Whey protein concentrate)	—	—
Ultragen	320	60 g (Dextrose)	20 g (Whey protien isolate)	—	4.5 g BCAA 6 g glutamine

exercise stimulates thirst. It goes without saying that it's hard to eat when you're not hungry and it's easy to drink when you're thirsty.

Drinks hydrate and nourish simultaneously. After a solid run workout you may need to drink more than 24 ounces of fluid to rehydrate, and you may need to consume 500 calories or more to take care of your immediate recovery nutrition needs. That's a lot of drinking and eating, if you choose to get your fluid from plain water and your energy from solid food. Recovery drinks allow you to satisfy your hydration and

Vitamins C & E	Electrolytes	Pros	Cons
100 mg C, 200 IU E	210 mg sodium 283 mg potassium 250 mg magnesium	Macronutrient balance; electrolyte content	None
60 mg C, 60 IU E	100 mg sodium 240 mg potassium 60 mg magnesium	High in key amino acids	Too much protein or fat; not enough carbs
470 mg C, 400 IU E	210 mg sodium 270 mg potassium 260 mg magnesium	Macronutrient balance; electrolyte content; high in vitamins C and E	None
—	110 mg sodium 64 mg potassium 128 mg magnesium	Good balance of hydration and nutrition	No vitamin C or E
—	250 mg sodium 10 mg potassium 16 mg magnesium	Good thirst quencher	Not enough carbs, protein, key amino acids, potassium, or magnesium; no vitamin C or E
400 mg C, 400 IU E	350 mg sodium 200 mg potassium 250 mg magnesium	Good macronutrient balance; very high in key amino acids, electrolytes, and vitamins C and E	None

nutrition needs from a single source that takes up less space in your stomach than a solid meal plus a lot of water.

Drinks are more convenient "on the run." When you work out away from home, whether it's speed intervals at the local high school track or a long trail run in the park, having a premixed squeeze bottle of recovery drink waiting for you in the car can prevent you from missing the recovery window. For that matter, even when you're at home, mixing up a recovery drink may seem infinitely less taxing than fixing a sit-down meal after you've just left it all out on the road in a hard training session.

Drinks work faster. Recovery drinks are usually absorbed through the gut faster than solid meals, for more than one reason. First, nutrient-containing liquids empty from the gut faster than solid foods, at least initially. (If stomach volume is kept high through subsequent drinking, the emptying rate remains high.) In addition, when you consume solids and liquids together, the body absorbs the liquids preferentially. So when you wash down a solid meal with water, your meal has to wait around in your stomach while the water is absorbed. Finally, the better recovery drinks are made with fast-acting nutrients such as high glycemic index carbohydrates and whey protein and contain small amounts of absorption-slowing ingredients such as fiber and fat. It's hard to come up with a solid-food meal that matches these characteristics.

Drinks are precisely formulated for recovery. In addition to being formulated for fast action, recovery drinks are also formulated to contain everything your body needs most during the acute recovery period and little that your body doesn't need right away. Again, natural foods just can't match this combination of virtues. For example, you'd have to eat a mountain of cheese to get the same amount of protein you'll get in a recovery drink containing whey protein isolate, but with cheese you'd also get an immense amount of fat, lactose, and overall calories.

NONNUTRITIONAL WAYS TO BOOST RECOVERY

Beyond resting and practicing proper recovery nutrition, there's not a lot you can do to boost recovery after workouts. Some of the things runners commonly do for the sake of boosting their recovery—including stretching, ice baths, massage, and taking pain relief medications—have been proven ineffective for this purpose in formal studies. (All of these measures can be effective in speeding injury recovery, however.) Only those measures that enhance the quality of your rest between workouts are able to boost your recovery. Sleep and stress management are the two nonnutritional factors that make the biggest difference in your recovery efforts.

Sleep is the closest thing to absolute rest and is invaluable to general health and recovery from running. Athletes who train rigorously require slightly more sleep than others. Insufficient sleep reduces the body's ability to process glucose, and therefore to produce energy. It also heightens levels of cortisol, the above-mentioned stress hormone that attacks muscle tissue and therefore must be suppressed in order for proper post-workout tissue repair to occur. In addition, human growth hormone, the muscle-building hormone that plays the biggest role in rebuilding tissue after exercise, requires sleep for full activation, so the less sleep you get, the less muscle you wake up with. Sleep loss also weakens the immune system by reducing the activity of interleukins, molecules involved in signaling between cells of the immune system.

As few as 30 hours of *cumulative* sleep deprivation have been shown to reduce the cardiovascular performance of runners by more than 10 percent. If you need 8 hours of sleep a night and only get 7, your running will be seriously compromised within a month. It is extremely important that you get all the sleep you need on a nightly basis. These strategies may help.

■ Figure out how much sleep you actually need. Monitor how long you typically sleep on weekends or during vacations. This is your benchmark for every night.

- Go to bed at the same time every night and get up at the same time every morning. This consistent routine will program your body to sleep when it's supposed to.
- Do relaxing things that prepare you for sleep during the last hour or two before your bedtime. Read a book, listen to quiet music, or have a pleasant conversation with your spouse.
- Create a sleep-friendly bedroom. It should be very dark, perfectly quiet (soft white noise is OK), and cool.

Stress management enhances the quality of your rest time between workouts and boosts your recovery. Stress inhibits exercise recovery by altering your hormonal environment in ways that slow down recovery processes such as the replenishment of muscle glycogen and the restoration of normal immune system function. Psychological stressors such as interpersonal conflicts and deadline pressure at work cause your adrenal glands to release high levels of adrenaline and cortisol that increase energy usage and reduce energy storage, increase muscle tension and muscle tissue breakdown, and suppress the immune system. The more stress you have in your life on any given day, the slower you will recover from training that day. If your stress level is high every day— well, then, you're in trouble. High stress levels have even been linked to higher injury rates in athletes, and especially in athletes with poor stress coping skills.

There are many effective ways to reduce the amount of psychological stress you experience. Here are a few.

- Remove unnecessary stressors from your life. If, for example, your work commute is a major stressor, move closer to your workplace, or find a job that's closer to home, or use flex-time to avoid heavy traffic hours, or telecommute (work from home) 1 or 2 days a week, if possible.
- Practice relaxation exercises. Here's a simple one: Find a quiet

space, lay down face up, relax all of your muscles, remove all thoughts from your mind, and focus on your breathing. For 15 minutes, inhale through your nose and exhale through your mouth.

■ Replace negative thoughts with positive ones. Get in the habit of paying attention to your own thoughts and catching negative thoughts early. Cut off these thoughts and replace them with more helpful ones. For example, if you find yourself worrying about an upcoming performance evaluation at work, stop this thought and say to yourself, "I am competent, and I give my best effort each day. If my supervisor is fair, she will recognize my value. If she's not fair—well, I can't control that, so there's no use fretting about it." Research shows that feelings of lacking control are major causes of stress. Learning to let go of such worries is one of the most powerful things you can do to reduce stress in your life.

■ Learn and practice better relationship skills. Interpersonal tension and conflict in familial, friendship, and business relationships is another common source of stress. This type of stress can be sharply reduced if you learn better ways to communicate with others. For example, showing empathy—that is, showing that you recognize the needs and feelings of others—in your communications is a great way to make your relationships more positive. Being honest (yet tactful) at all times is also important in this regard.

■ Find time for things you enjoy. The experience of pleasure is a terrific stress buster. Don't let a day go by without indulging in an activity that you enjoy, whether it's reading, listening to music, cooking, talking to your best friend on the phone—or running!

CHAPTER 8

EATING RIGHT NOW

Eating "on the run" has become the norm in our society. We eat fewer home-cooked meals than ever before. The phenomenon of a complete nuclear family sitting down at the same table at the same time to share a meal is on its way to extinction. Office workers take fewer formal lunch breaks and instead eat while working at their desks. Not only do we spend less time planning and preparing meals, but we also spend less time actually eating (which is not to say we're eating less). We miss or skip more breakfasts, lunches, and dinners and get a greater share of our daily calories from spontaneous snacks and meal replacements. Eating while driving is more common than ever before. Some experts even suggest that we eat more meals standing up than in the past.

Meanwhile, the overall quality of our diet is at an all-time low. Is there a connection here? Yes, there is. But it's not that the fastest and most convenient foods are inherently unhealthy. It's certainly true that the most accessible foods away from home tend to come from fast-food restaurants and convenience stores, and that most of these foods are unhealthy. If, for example, you find yourself at an airport, and feeling hungry, you may have to search high and low to uncover a (relatively) healthy meal option. If you're taking a summer road trip, the challenge of finding wholesome foods at a highway rest stop might be even greater. And if your stomach begins to rumble while you're attending a major sporting event at a stadium or arena, you'll probably find no healthy options whatsoever at the concession stands. Likewise, a lot of the meals that require the least preparation time at home are highly processed prepared foods (boxed macaroni and cheese, for example) that aren't very healthy, either.

Nevertheless, eating healthily is not necessarily less convenient or more time consuming than eating poorly. An apple, for example, is quite healthy, requires little preparation time, and travels well. Beyond the speed and convenience factors, there are two other major explanations for the connection between eating on the run and eating poorly. One is the simple fact that we prefer the taste of less healthy foods that also happen to be fast and convenient. As I explained earlier, nature has endowed us with a double-edged preference for energy-dense foods, and modern food technology has given us unprecedented opportunity to indulge this preference. A cheeseburger is not inherently faster or more convenient than a salad, but we tend to choose cheeseburgers over salads because cheeseburgers are more energy-dense and consequently more palatable to most people.

Another reason for the connection between eating on the run and eating poorly is what we might call the conformity factor. Whether we want to believe it or not, we humans tend to unconsciously obey the dominant messages of society and to blindly conform to the habits of those around us. The vast majority of corporate advertising dollars in the food sector are spent on foods (and beverages) that aren't very healthy. Less than 2 percent of food-related advertising money is used to sell fruits, vegetables, and grains combined. The fact that most of our friends, relatives, and co-workers are influenced by "junk" food advertising only increases its influence over us. When everyone else wants to go out for cheeseburgers, it's hard to play the spoiler who would rather get a salad.

Given all of these forces that encourage us to eat poorly when we wish to eat in a convenient and time-efficient manner, is it really possible to eat better without sacrificing convenience and efficiency? Of course it is. All it requires is that you learn and consistently practice a few basic strategies. The objective of this chapter is to teach you these strategies so you can eat right—now!

STRATEGIES FOR EATING OUT

Studies indicate that people who eat out more often tend to eat more fat, more total calories, and less fiber than those who eat out less often. One study that tracked the dining out habits of more than 3,000 men and women for 15 years found those who ate at fast-food restaurants more than twice a week gained 10 pounds more and experienced a twofold greater increase in insulin resistance (a type 2 diabetes risk factor) than those who ate at fast-food restaurants less than once a week.

Based on these data, many dietitians advise their clients to eat out less often. It's certainly not bad advice insofar as it is realistic. With just a little effort, for example, you can create a habit of preparing healthy lunches at home and taking them to work instead of eating at fried chicken, taco, and hamburger joints near your workplace every noon hour. But avoiding restaurants is not always possible. Some of us travel a lot and have no choice but to eat often at restaurants. Some of us are involved in frequent, restaurant-based working lunches, and to miss these would compromise our work. And some of us are so busy, overburdened, stressed out, and frazzled that we just need to cut ourselves some slack and have others prepare and serve our food more often than we prepare it for ourselves. That's OK. I've been there.

No matter how frequently or infrequently you eat out, it's good to know how to eat healthily at restaurants. Following are a few simple tips that will help you in this regard.

Choose restaurants with healthier options. All restaurants are not equal in terms of the availability of healthy menu items. If you're serious about eating well when eating out, don't paint yourself into a corner by going to restaurants that don't offer healthy menu items you can enjoy.

The typical fast-food hamburger restaurant has almost nothing wholesome to offer. Under pressure from various sources, some of the major chains have begun making halfhearted efforts to introduce menu items that are not as egregiously bad as the rest, but so far these efforts have not amounted to much. Real, fresh vegetables and fruits (french fries and ketchup don't count) remain exceedingly rare at a majority of these establishments. For this reason, I advise you to simply avoid McDonald's, Kentucky Fried Chicken, and the like except on rare occasions. If and when you do find yourself at such a place, ask your server for written nutrition information before ordering. You can also research the nutrition content of any major chain's menu items ahead of time by visiting the company's official Web site or by purchasing a copy of a book such as *The Complete Book of Food Counts*.

There are plenty of restaurants—even inexpensive restaurants with fast service—where it's not at all difficult to get a wholesome meal. Delis and sandwich shops, Chinese, Japanese, and Mexican restaurants, salad bars, smoothie joints, and buffets are among the types of restaurants that can usually feed you quickly and cheaply without clogging your arteries with trans fats. A simple guideline to use when choosing where to eat out is the vegetable rule. If a given restaurant has one or more real, honest-to-goodness vegetable items (for example, salads not made with iceberg lettuce, which contains virtually no nutrition), it's probably OK. Potatoes and vegetables compromised by their manner of preparation (for example, creamed spinach) don't count as real and honest-to-goodness.

Order the healthier options. Choosing a restaurant with healthy menu options doesn't do you any good unless you actually order them. In deciding what to order from a restaurant menu, follow the same four principles of healthy eating that were discussed in Chapter 2, and especially the first two: eat natural foods, and eat a balance and variety of foods.

The two simplest ways to eat more naturally at restaurants are to avoid fried foods (except stir fries) and to either avoid or strictly limit desserts. Fried foods, as we have seen, are quite "unnatural" in that frying greatly increases the caloric density of foods and damages some of the oils used. Restaurant menus tend to be full of fried foods. Instead, go for menu items that are baked, boiled, grilled, poached, roasted, steamed, or stir-fried. The processing that produces our favorite desserts also results in foods that are unnaturally dense calorically and unnaturally empty nutritionally. I won't go as far as to tell you to never eat desserts at restaurants, but I do suggest that you eat them seldom, or eat just a few bites to satisfy your sweet tooth.

The two simplest ways to eat more balanced meals at restaurants are to avoid fat-heavy items and to always order vegetables. Restaurant offerings tend to be seriously unbalanced in the direction of fat. You can improve the nutritional balance of your restaurant meals by avoiding or going light on fatty sauces, salad dressings, and dairy foods. On some menus, low-fat menu items are identified as such (often with a heart icon, courtesy of the American Heart Association). Another effective way to improve the nutritional balance of your restaurant meals is to make sure you order vegetables. It's all too easy to walk out of a restaurant without having eaten real, honest-to-goodness vegetables. Prioritizing them when you order will not only increase the

(continued on page 170)

SMART RESTAURANT CHOICES

The accompanying table will help guide you toward the healthiest menu choices at various types of restaurants. The middle column lists menu items that are more balanced and good choices. The last column lists popular

AT . . .	ORDER THIS . . .	NOT THIS . . .
Breakfast	Egg and vegetable scramble	Ham and cheese omelet
	Egg white/egg substitute omelet (with vegetables)	Pork sausage
		Corned beef hash
	Fresh fruit/fruit juice	Bacon
	Oatmeal	
	Pancakes (w/o butter)	
A Chinese restaurant	Steamed rice (with all entrées)	Sweet and sour chicken
	Beef, chicken, or shrimp with broccoli	Egg fu young
	Moo shu shrimp/chicken	General Tso's chicken
	Stir-fried vegetables (with tofu)	
A fast-food joint	Chicken breast sandwich	Cheeseburger
	Garden salad	French fries
	Fruit bowl	Onion rings
		Soft drink
An Indian restaurant	Rice pilaf	Chicken korma
	Tandoori chicken or shrimp	Onion bhaji
	Beef, chicken, or fish vindaloo	Samosa
	Vegetable curry	

choices that should be limited to special occasions, as they are high in saturated fat and sometimes trans fats as well.

AT . . .	ORDER THIS . . .	NOT THIS . . .
An Italian restaurant	Any pasta Marinara sauce Primavera sauce	Meat- or cheese-stuffed ravioli Veal parmesan Lasagna
A Mexican restaurant	Black bean soup Burrito (beef, chicken, fish, shrimp, or vegetable) Fajitas (chicken, shrimp, or vegetable) Taco (chicken or fish) Guacamole *And remember: hold the cheese and sour cream*	Fried fish taco Quesadilla Burrito with "the works" Chorizo Cheese and sour cream
A deli	Whole wheat bread (with all sandwiches) Chicken breast Grilled vegetables Lean roast beef Turkey breast *And remember: hold the cheese and mayonnaise*	Any sandwich with white bread Meatball sub Reuben sandwich BLT

amount of quality nutrients in your meals but will also reduce the amount of bad stuff you eat by leaving less room for it in your stomach. It's easy enough to ask if your entrée comes with vegetables. If it doesn't, order one or two steamed vegetables as a side dish, or order a salad as an appetizer with the dressing on the side.

Don't be afraid to make special requests. There are two distinct types of restaurant patrons. On the one hand there are the "Sallys"—named after Meg Ryan's character in the film *When Harry Met Sally*—who are not afraid to completely disregard the menu and order exactly what they want, exactly the way they want it, no matter how much trouble it causes the cooking staff. On the other hand, there are diners who tend to view the restaurant staff as though they were their hosts in a private home and are therefore afraid to make any special requests. When it comes to eating healthily in restaurants, it's much better to be a Sally.

First of all, if you have any questions—about how a particular menu item is prepared, about alternatives to listed menu items, or whatever else—open your mouth and ask. For example, if you would like to order an omelet made with egg substitutes—even though this option is not listed on the menu—don't assume egg substitutes are not available. Find out. Also, be bold in collaborating with your server and/or chef to come up with a healthier version of whatever you wish to order, whether that means replacing a meat sauce with a meatless one, holding the cheese, substituting brown rice for potatoes, or something else entirely. In my experience, most restaurants are happy to do what it takes to please you.

Mind the drinks. At restaurants we tend to drink larger quantities of beverages and/or indulge in beverages that we don't drink at home (soft drinks, cocktails, and so forth). This tendency can unnecessarily inflate the number of calories we consume in restaurant meals. A pint of draft beer contains about 230 calories. A medium Coca-Cola at Burger King contains 260 calories. That's about 10 percent of a typical runner's daily energy needs in one cup.

Water is one good alternative to high-calorie restaurant beverages, but not the only one. Others include herbal tea with lemon or a little honey, lightly sweetened homemade iced tea, and sparkling water. At many fast-food restaurants there are no healthy drink options besides tap water. That's another reason to shy away from fast-food restaurants. When you do find yourself in such a place, avoid ordering the "meal combos" that come with a soft drink. Order à la carte instead and choose water as your beverage.

Don't get your money's worth. Because eating at a restaurant is usually more expensive than eating at home, we often adopt a get-my-money's-worth attitude at restaurants that can result in our eating much more than we need to. This is especially tempting in buffet restaurants, but it's also a problem at other restaurants that serve large portions. You must not feel obligated to "clean your plate." Try to eat the same amount you eat when you control your own portions at home. Employ the 1-to-5 scale of fullness described in Chapter 4 and stop eating when you hit level 3 or 4. Feel free to ask your server about portion sizes before you order and to request a smaller-than-normal serving when the standard portion size seems too large.

SMART SHOPPING STRATEGIES

The place where you have the most control over what you eat is home. But the nutrition you get at home is only as good as the choices you make at the supermarket and grocery store. Here are some tips to make your grocery shopping more supportive of your performance nutrition agenda—and more efficient, to better fit your busy lifestyle.

Be selective in where you shop. Don't automatically do all of your grocery shopping at the supermarket that's nearest to your home. While that sort of convenience is valuable, it is not the only factor worth considering. For example, the supermarket that's closest to my home is somewhat small, offers a mediocre selection, has a below-average produce department, and is usually crowded, so that the time I save in driving there is lost in the checkout line. I shopped there once, when I was new to the neighborhood, and never went back.

Besides proximity, here are some other qualities I recommend looking for in a grocery store or supermarket:

- A pleasant environment and good service. Shopping is a chore that few savor, but if you want to eat well you need to shop well. You will be more likely to take your time and shop well if the overall shopping experience in a particular store is pleasant.
- Excellent variety. If a particular store has everything, it spares you the need to shop at more than one place.
- An emphasis on healthy foods, or at least a good health foods section. Health food grocery stores such as Whole Foods and Trader Joe's are spreading rapidly throughout the country. They aren't the least expensive stores, but they are the places where you're most likely to find an abundance of organic foods, healthy prepared foods, and so forth. There are also plenty of regular supermarkets that cater to a more health-conscious customer base, but many others do not. Learn to tell the difference (for example, how many organic fruits and vegetables are available?).
- A great produce section. Fresh fruits and vegetables are the most important foods in your diet, and your supermarket or grocery store should reflect that fact. The produce section should be large and loaded with variety; the fruits and vegeta-

bles should be of high quality, and there should be plenty of organic stuff.

What about price? Your budget is your budget, but I believe that food is the last part of your budget where you should cut corners. Drive a car with better gas mileage, switch to a cheaper cable television package—do what you have to do so that "money is no object" when it comes to food buying.

Start with staples. Food shopping seems a lesser hassle when you divide food into two categories: staples and nonstaples. Staples are healthy foods that you eat frequently. Mine include oatmeal, whole wheat bread, bananas, rice, pasta, and fish. When you consciously label your staples as such, you realize the list really isn't that long, and you also realize what you could (and in some cases should) do without (ice cream, snack chips, etc.). Make the staples your top priority on every trip to the grocery store or supermarket.

Read labels. Know what to look for—and what to look out for—on ingredients labels. Here are some simple guidelines:

- Saturated fat: The less the better
- Trans fat: The less the better
- Fiber: The more the better
- Sugar: The less added sugar the better (usually listed as sucrose, corn syrup, or high fructose corn syrup)
- Juices: 100% juice
- Baked goods: Whole grains (e.g., "100% whole wheat")
- Sodium: The less the better

Also make an effort to choose products without artificial sweeteners (especially aspartame), artificial colorings (especially red dye No. 40, blue dye No. 1, and yellow dye No. 5, aka tartrazine), and preservatives (especially nitrites) listed among their ingredients. All of these additives are associated with negative health effects and are banned in some countries outside the United States.

It's usually very easy to distinguish healthier, more natural packaged foods from less healthy and natural foods.

Don't be afraid of frozen. In relation to food, the word "frozen" connotes unhealthiness in the minds of many shoppers, but the reputation is not always justified. Some frozen foods are as healthy as their nonfrozen counterparts while having the added advantages of resistance to spoilage and, in many cases, easier preparation.

Frozen fruits and vegetables are often even more nutritious than their "fresh" counterparts (except in the case of organic fresh fruits and vegetables). This is because most frozen fruits and vegetables are actually frozen fresh, whereas these days many "fresh" fruits and vegetables are stored for weeks or even months under conditions that prevent ripening and lower their nutrient content.

While a majority of frozen entrées and other frozen prepared foods (pizzas and so forth) are high in sodium and fat and low in certain vitamins and minerals, there are some healthy frozen prepared foods. These include some veggie burgers, fish entrées, pastas and pierogies, burritos and wraps, stir-fry bowls, and various soy products. My favorite supermarket has a special freezer section containing only organic and healthier frozen items, which makes it easier to find them, but even in stores that lack this convenience you can find them without too much trouble by following the label guidelines listed above.

Stock up. The more food you buy when you buy groceries, the less often you have to shop and the more time you have to do other things. Of course, you can't really stock up on certain perishable foods such as fresh vegetables, and there are many nonperishable foods that you'll want to avoid. But there are also a lot of healthy staples and other foods that you can buy in quantities sufficient to last several weeks. Among them are rice, pasta, oatmeal and breakfast cereal, dried beans, and the various healthy frozen foods mentioned above.

I do two distinct types of grocery shopping. The first type is the major shopping trip, in which I load up on nonperishable foods and also buy any perishable foods (fresh vegetables, meats, fresh seafood, etc.) I may need. I make these trips once every 2 or 3 weeks. Between them I do quick trips, wherein I pick up only the perishable foods I need. This system works well to minimize the total amount of my life I spend cruising the aisles of supermarkets.

Another simple way to achieve this end is to keep a running list of grocery needs at home. Whenever you run out of something or think of an item you need, add it to the list. When you're ready to shop, take the list with you. This will minimize those annoying trips to buy one or two items you forgot.

THE ART OF SNACKING

Skipping meals and not eating for long stretches of time during the day are common problems among busy working people. Commuting, meetings, phone calls, deadlines, and stuffed inboxes make it all too easy to go several hours without eating. The problem is not just that such activities leave little time for eating but also that they distract you from your hunger. Some people have a perverse tendency to derive satisfaction from not eating, which only exacerbates this problem. I'm not talking about an outright eating disorder; I'm talking about a very widespread penchant to associate eating itself with weight gain. The irony, of course, is that men and women who eat infrequently are more likely to be overweight because they often overeat and make poor food choices when they do get around to eating.

Developing a healthy snacking habit is a great way to break out of this trap. By making healthy snacks a part of your daily eating patterns, you will be more likely to balance your energy intake with your actual energy needs and also to get more overall nutrition. As a result, you will find it easier to maintain a healthy weight and you will also perform better at work and as a runner. Following are four simple guidelines for healthy snacking.

Eat snacks that are both nutritious and delicious. We often associate snacking with indulging in tasty but unwholesome treats such as potato chips and candy bars. This is not the sort of snacking I recommend. Your needs will be much better served if you snack on foods that supply nutrients we Americans tend to get too little of (e.g., phytonutrients, which are the nonessential but extremely healthful nutrients in plants) rather than too much of (saturated fat).

This is not to say that your snacks need not be tasty. With rare exceptions, you should enjoy everything you eat and eat only what you enjoy. There are dozens of healthy snack options, at least a few of which you will like enough to look forward to eating. It's important that you build your snacking habit on these foods, or it probably won't remain a habit very long. See the "Five Healthy Snacks" section of this chapter (beginning on page 178) for some examples of snacks that are as delicious as they are nutritious.

Have snacks handy when you need them. If you normally spend many hours of the day away from home, and especially if you travel a lot, find simple ways to take snacks with you and make it second nature to do so every time you leave home. Devote a special compartment of your briefcase, carry-on bag, or book bag to serve as a snack holder. As soon as you eat the snack that's in there, replace it with a fresh one.

You can also stash snacks in your vehicle. I usually keep some snack bars in a storage compartment located between the front seats of my car. Just beware of extremes in temperature and the effects they might have on particular snack types. For example, most fresh fruits hold up better than dried fruits in cold weather, while the opposite is true in the summer heat.

Another obvious place to keep snacks handy is at your workplace, in a desk drawer, a locker, or another out-of-the-way spot. It goes without saying that all such snacks should be wholesome and therefore provide a better alternative to the types of snacks that are commonly available in most work environments (doughnuts, snack machine fare, and so forth).

Snack consciously and purposefully. All too often, we snack opportunistically and even unconsciously, without a thought as to whether the snack we're eating provides valuable nutrition and needed energy. Generally, a snack makes sense if, and only if, it is nutrient-dense and eaten at a time when its energy content can be put to good use. Eating a doughnut at the office an hour after breakfast just because a co-worker happened to arrive with a box of Krispy Kremes is not an example of conscious and purposeful snacking. Eating an orange at your desk at midmorning to keep your energy up until lunchtime is an example of conscious and purposeful snacking.

Don't oversnack. Almost by definition, snacks are meant to be small. Snacking works best to moderate your overall caloric intake during the day if you eat one to three small snacks throughout the day (a single piece of fruit, a couple of handfuls of nuts) in addition to moderate-size meals (i.e., meals that are slightly smaller than they would be if you did not snack). If you eat large snacks in addition to normal meals, the overall effect of your snack will be only to inflate your daily caloric intake.

FIVE HEALTHY SNACKS FOR RUNNERS

A good snack must have three essential characteristics: It must be wholesome, tasty, and convenient. Many snack choices meet these three criteria. But none offer a better combination of wholesomeness, tastiness, and convenience than the following five.

ENERGY BAR

Compact and individually wrapped, energy bars (and healthy snack bars) travel better than just about any other kind of snack. You can toss a few in an airplane carry-on bag and stuff your bag in an overhead bin without fearing that your snacks will be ruined, as a banana surely would be.

The best energy bars for snacking are not the same as the best energy bars for pre-exercise use. The ideal pre-exercise bar is high in carbs and low in just about everything else. For general snacking, it's better to eat a bar with a more even balance of macro nutrients and fiber, as it will quell your hunger longer and give you more lasting energy. Best of all are those few energy bars that are made with whole foods (brown rice, cranberries, dates, oats, raisins, etc.) because they are highly nutrient-dense.

Examples of good energy bars for snacking are the Aloha Energy Bar and the Fruit & Nut Delight by Be Natural.

SOUP CUP

When you want a hot snack, and you have access to a microwave oven or a stovetop and teakettle, a soup cup can be just the thing. These dehydrated soup mixes are eaten in the packaging they're sold in—just add water and grab a spoon.

Some brands are healthier than others. Choose those that are lower in salt and have a shorter list of ingredients (which usually indicates fewer unnatural additives). Vegetable- and bean-based soup cups such as lentil and vegetable minestrone tend to be the most nutrient-dense. Nile Spice makes several healthy and delicious soup cups, including a yummy lentil curry couscous soup.

My favorite soup cup for runners: Black bean. Hearty and satisfying, this soup is an excellent source of protein, fiber, and various minerals including iron and manganese.

FRESH FRUIT

If, like most Americans, you are currently not eating enough fruit (fewer than 4 servings a day), you might want to consider making fresh fruit your primary snack option. In addition to being healthy and tasty, many types of fruit travel well and require little or no preparation. Apples and pears fare particularly well on the road. Another option is a fruit cup containing a medley of fruits such as grapes, strawberries, and sliced pineapple, cantaloupe, and watermelon. You can find freshly prepared fruit cups at many supermarkets.

My favorite fruit for runners: Organic strawberries. They're sweet, succulent, flavorful, and rich in vitamin C, iron, fiber, folic acid, and antioxidant phytonutrients.

SMOOTHIE

My personal favorite snacks are fruit smoothies. I blend my own smoothies at home every morning at about 10 o'clock, smack between breakfast and lunch. In addition to providing three or four complete servings of fruit, my homemade smoothies provide a ton of additional stuff thanks to the additions I like to blend in. These include spirulina (a microalgae rich in protein, beta-carotene, vitamin B_{12}, iron, and the essential fatty acid GLA—gamma linolenic acid), aloe vera juice (which promotes body tissue healing), noni juice (nutrient-rich juice derived from a Polynesian fruit), creatine powder (a muscle builder), flax oil (rich in omega-3 fatty acids), or powdered vitamins and minerals. I could practically live on these super beverages.

If you don't have access to a blender in the middle of the day, there are two other ways to snack on smoothies. First, there are smoothie restaurants (Jamba Juice, Smoothie King, etc.) popping up all across the country these days. If there's one in the vicinity of your workplace, go there! In addition, there are some excellent bottled smoothies, made by the likes of Odwalla and Naked, which are available at many grocery and health food stores. Stash these in your office refrigerator.

Bear in mind that smoothies tend to be rather energy-dense. For example, a Smoothie King Cranberry Supreme smoothie contains 577 calories. That's almost a meal. The calories you get from most smoothies are quality calories, but you still need to figure them into your total daily energy requirement.

My favorite smoothie for runners: This smoothie offers three full servings of fruit, along with all of the vitamins, minerals, and phytonutrients these fruits contain, as well as plenty of carbohydrates to fuel your next run.

Mix the following ingredients in a blender:

8 ounces orange juice
4 ounces vanilla nonfat yogurt
1 medium banana
3 ounces frozen strawberries
3 ounces frozen blueberries

Nondairy version: replace yogurt with ice

TRAIL MIX

Trail mix is another snack that combines the virtues of wholesomeness, tastiness, and convenience. There are many varieties of trail mix. Standard ingredients include peanuts, cashews, and other nuts, sunflower seeds, raisins, dried cranberries and other dried fruits, and coconut flakes. Sweet-tooth versions also contain such things as chocolate chips, M&M's, and yogurt-covered raisins. Stick with the all-natural trail mixes, except for the occasional treat.

Like smoothies, trail mixes tend to pack a lot of calories. For example, just one quarter-cup of Northwest Delights Nooksack Trail Mix contains 110 calories. All of these calories come from nutritious whole foods (peanuts, raisins, dried pineapple, and papaya), but they still count against your total daily requirement, so it's best to keep your trail mix snacks fairly small.

My favorite trail mix for runners: All-natural trail mix containing dark raisins, golden raisins, dried apricots, and walnut slivers. Heavy on the fruit, this mix has fewer calories than most trail mixes but is no less tasty.

FAST AND HEALTHY DINNERS

Theoretically, it is possible to maintain a healthy diet without ever cooking. In fact, a good friend of mine, who's bursting with health and is an excellent runner, never cooks. But he's also single and lives in an urban environment that is teeming with inexpensive ethnic restaurants that offer some wholesome menu items. In other words, his situation is exceptional; yet even he would save money and perhaps even some time, while nourishing himself still better than he already does, if he learned to cook a few fast and healthy dinners.

The desire to spare precious time and energy is the reason most men and women cite for cooking rarely or never (or for eating the same dinner every night, as I did in my first year after college). However, there are healthy dinners you can prepare in the same amount of time and with the same amount of effort it takes to swing by a Chinese restaurant for takeout on the way home from work. Developing a small repertoire of healthy and easy-to-prepare dinner menus will allow you to take greater control over your diet, so you can truly optimize your performance nutrition through foods you enjoy eating. For example, important foods such as whole grains can be hard to come by in restaurants but are easy to incorporate into delicious home-cooked meals. By and large, preparing your own dinners is also more economical than eating out.

If you don't do much cooking, a good initial goal to shoot for is a repertoire of seven dinner menus: one for each day of the week. This will give you the variety you need for optimal performance nutrition and to avoid becoming bored with your evening meal. Here are seven dinner ideas for optimal running performance. All are low in saturated fat and high in quality proteins and low glycemic index carbs. Be sure to include a steamed vegetable or salad where recommended for the rich assortment of vitamins, minerals, and fiber these "side items" offer.

MONDAY: STIR-FRY

Buy some precooked brown rice (e.g., Success Brown Rice) and prepare according to package instructions (5 minutes). Heat some olive oil in a stir-fry pan. Add vegetables of your choice to the pan. Popular options are snow peas, broccoli tips, baby carrots, baby corn, mushrooms, baby bok choy, bell peppers, onions, and bean sprouts. For maximum convenience, you can buy and use a package of fresh or frozen stir-fry vegetables. Also add scallops, shrimp, or slices of chicken breast, beef, or tofu. Season with a packet of Kikkoman Fried Rice Seasoning Mix or something similar. Cook the mixture for 5 to 7 minutes over medium heat and serve over the rice.

TUESDAY: SALMON

Buy a jar of gourmet salsa (such as Guzman's Peach Salsa) and a *wild* salmon fillet (wild salmon is much higher in omega-3 fatty acids than farmed salmon). If you can't find wild salmon in the seafood department of your supermarket, check the freezer section. Preheat the oven broiler. Spread a little olive oil on a baking sheet, sprinkle salt and pepper on both sides of the fillet, and place it on the baking sheet. Broil for about 10 minutes. When it's done, spread some salsa on top of it and serve with brown rice and steamed vegetables or a salad.

WEDNESDAY: MEXICAN WRAP

Sauté some diced onions in olive oil. Add some lean ground turkey and brown it. When it's halfway browned, add black beans from a can, precooked brown rice, and diced tomatoes. Warm a whole wheat or whole kernel corn tortilla in the oven, then put it on a plate. Spoon some of the turkey mixture onto the middle of the tortilla, top it with a little grated Monterey Jack cheese, and fold it fajita-style. Serve with a steamed vegetable or green salad.

THURSDAY: HAMBURGER

Buy some lean ground beef—or better yet, some grass-fed organic beef, if you can get your hands on it. Sprinkle some steak seasoning on it and shape it into hamburger patties. Fire up the grill and grill the patties the way you like them, or fry them in a little olive oil on medium heat, 3 to 4 minutes per side. Serve on a whole-wheat bun and top with lettuce, onion, tomato, pickles, ketchup, and/or mustard. Round out the meal with a steamed vegetable or green salad.

FRIDAY: TUNA STEAKS

Buy a bottle of seafood marinade and marinate some ahi tuna steaks in it according to instructions on the bottle. Pour a little olive oil into a skillet and place it over medium heat. Remove the tuna steaks from the marinade and cook them for 4 to 5 minutes per side. Serve with rice and a vegetable or salad.

SATURDAY: DIJON CHICKEN BREASTS

Place some boneless, skinless chicken breasts in an ovenproof casserole dish. In a small bowl, mix equal amounts of light sour cream and Dijon mustard. Preheat the oven to 350°F. Sprinkle a little seasoning salt on the chicken breasts and then cover them with the mustard/sour cream mixture. Bake for 35 to 40 minutes. Serve with rice and a vegetable or salad.

SUNDAY: SPAGHETTI AND TOMATO SAUCE WITH SAUSAGE

Boil whole wheat spaghetti according to package directions. Warm your favorite jarred pasta sauce (I like the Newman's Own line) in a saucepot. Slice some precooked Italian sausage or tofu mock sausage and add to the sauce. Strain the spaghetti when it's ready and top with the sauce. Serve with a garden salad.

CHAPTER 9

CHOOSING THE RIGHT SUPPLEMENTS

The next time you have a dietary supplement bottle within reach, take a look at the back label. You will probably see some benefit claims followed by an asterisk that leads you to the following phrase: "These statements have not been evaluated by the Food and Drug Administration." This caveat sums up the challenge we face in choosing the right supplements (if any) to use for the sake of optimizing performance nutrition. There are dozens of different types of dietary supplements on the market. There is also a lot of available information about these supplements. But most of the available information—such as the benefit claims on product labels—comes from the companies that make the supplements. There's a word for this type of information: advertising.

Fortunately, although it is in the minority, and not as accessible, there is also objective information about the effects of dietary supplements. Most of this information comes from university laboratories that conduct formal, clinical trials to test the effects of promising supplements. In fact, supplement makers seldom put a new supplement on the market without first seeing some evidence of a benefit revealed in a clinical trial. Yet even the information about supplements that comes out of university laboratories is not always objective. Consider the example of Beta-hydroxy-beta-methylbutyrate (HMB), a compound that became very popular as a muscle-building supplement several years ago after one researcher discovered that it produced amazing results in strength athletes. The only problem was that the researcher who performed these studies also owned a supplements company that sold HMB, and subsequent research conducted by others found this particular supplement to be utterly useless.

It's also true that even when supplement research is done with the best of intentions, it can be faulty. For example, many studies designed to test the ergogenic (i.e., energy-boosting) effects of a supplement use an unreliable fixed-intensity format. In this format, subjects exercise (usually on stationary bikes) at a predetermined percentage of their individual VO_2max until they reach "voluntary exhaustion"—that is, until they decide they are too tired to continue at that intensity and quit. This format is known to have a low degree of reproducibility, which means that the results tend to vary widely when the test is repeated with the same subjects. The fixed-intensity format also tends to exaggerate the effects of the variable under scrutiny. When a true time trial format is used instead of a fixed-intensity format—in other words, when subjects cover a fixed distance as fast as they can, as in a real race—the effects tend to be more muted, and also more consistent. Yet many scientists continue to prefer using a fixed-intensity format precisely because they feel the exaggerated effects make differences "clearer."

So, if you can't trust advertising at all, and you never know when you can trust science, just what information concerning dietary supplements can you trust? The answer to this question is that you *can* trust science, but you have to trust it in the way that good scientists themselves trust it. A good scientist never puts too much faith in a

WHAT'S REALLY IN THE BOTTLE?

Unfortunately, dietary supplements often do not contain exactly what their labels claim they do. The most common problem is a discrepancy in the amount of the main active ingredient. One study that examined ephedra supplements (before they were banned) found that half of the products tested contained at least 20 percent more or less (usually less) ephedra than claimed, and one product contained none whatsoever!

The reason for such discrepancies is not always fraud. Sometimes it's just poor quality control that causes the ingredients to vary even among batches of the same brand of supplement. It is also not uncommon for supplements to contain ingredients that are not even listed on the label (a major concern for drug-tested elite athletes). In addition, a variety of other ingredient quality problems are frequently seen.

There are plenty of dietary supplement manufacturers that hold themselves to the highest standards of integrity and quality control, and I strongly recommend that you buy your supplements from only these companies. But how can you distinguish them from the others? One way is to take out a subscription to ConsumerLab.com (www.consumerlab.com), an outfit whose sole mission is to assess the quality of supplements through independent laboratory testing. A 1-year online subscription costs only $24 and gives you access to thousands of test results. If you prefer paper, you can order a copy of the company's book, *ConsumerLab.com's Guide to Buying Vitamins and Supplements*.

single experiment, especially if it's the first of its kind (e.g., the first test of a certain supplement). Scientific truth is never an instant result of a single test but is always a balance of evidence that accumulates over time. Not even the best-designed experiment can reveal the whole truth about its object of inquiry. When evaluating any supplement, scientists need to approach it from a variety of angles and see definite trends emerge before they are able to draw firm conclusions.

The history of dietary supplements is littered with examples of individual supplements that seemed very promising in preliminary research but that ultimately turned out to be busts in one way or another. In each of these cases, manufacturers stoked the early hype and consumers got caught up in it, while good scientists contained their irrational exuberance, continued to scrutinize the supplement in question, and eventually uncovered the whole truth. You'll spare yourself a lot of money and disappointment, and possibly even some unpleasant side effects, if you ignore the hype and only use supplements whose benefits have been substantiated over time.

Having said that, I now must add that no dietary supplement has been shown to directly benefit the performance of all runners to a "must-have" degree. It's always more complicated than that. The few supplements that do have established benefits affect the performance of runners only indirectly. Some supplements are beneficial only in certain conditions. And it's always the case that individual runners are affected differently by the same supplement. For this reason, the process of testing a supplement is never completed in the laboratory; rather, it's not completed until you've given it a try and seen what it does (or does not do) for you.

In this chapter, I will tell you about 12 of the dietary supplements that are most relevant to runners. You'll learn their true effects, whether I recommend them, and how you should use them if you choose to try them.

CAFFEINE

In Chapter 6, I recommended that you take a caffeine supplement 30 to 60 minutes before racing because caffeine has a proven ergogenic effect. Specifically, it boosts endurance performance by reducing perceived effort and delaying nervous system fatigue. For the same reason, you might want to take caffeine before some of your tougher workouts. Doing so will likely allow you to perform 1 to 5 percent better in these workouts, derive a very slightly stronger training effect from them, and run a few ticks faster in your next race.

If you're a regular coffee or green tea drinker, then you're already taking a de facto pre-workout caffeine supplement (unless, of course, you drink your coffee or tea after you work out). While the ergogenic effect of caffeine is muted by habitual caffeine use, and may be stronger when it's taken in a pill instead of coffee or tea, caffeine still has a measurable effect on exercise performance when taken in a beverage by regular caffeine users.

The effect is greatest when the workout follows within an hour of caffeine intake and peters out after 5 or 6 hours, depending on the dosage. For this reason, if you are a morning coffee drinker, and you usually work out in the evening, you might consider moving your workout to the morning—after your coffee—at least on days when you have a tough workout planned.

Noncaffeine users who are serious about their running might choose to drink an espresso or take a caffeine pill perhaps once a week before their most challenging workouts. In addition to helping you get just a bit more out of your toughest workouts, it will also get you accustomed to running hard with caffeine in your body, which is certainly beneficial if you intend to use caffeine before races.

If you consciously avoid using caffeine for any reason, it's probably not worth starting to use it just for the sake of the small boost it will give you in your tougher workouts. For example, some people just don't react well to caffeine use; it makes them feel tense and jittery even in relatively small doses. Runners with this type of sensitivity are better off avoiding caffeine even before races.

In moderation, caffeine consumption does not cause any health problems. However, heavy caffeine use can cause or exacerbate problems ranging from headache to insomnia, and it is possible to become physically dependent on the drug. Caffeine is especially harmful when used as a means to stimulate artificial wakefulness or energy in those suffering from conditions such as chronic fatigue. So, if you do like caffeine, limit yourself to one mug of coffee or green tea in the morning. Those who rely on regular "caffeine injections" throughout the day are well advised to cut back.

The ergogenic effect of caffeine is dose-dependent. The maximum effect is seen with doses of 5 to 6 milligrams per kilogram of body weight. For a 150-pound runner this translates to roughly 340 to 400 milligrams, or the amount of caffeine you'd get in 14 to 17 ounces of drip-brewed coffee. The minimum amount of caffeine the average runner must consume for a measurable ergogenic effect is about 2 milligrams per kilogram of body weight. I recommend that you take the dose required for the maximum effect before races, but not every day. An average mug of drip-brewed coffee contains about 250 milligrams of caffeine, and that's plenty on typical training days.

CARNITINE

A natural compound with properties resembling both vitamins and amino acids, carnitine (also known as L-carnitine) is supplied in the diet by meats and is also manufactured by the body in the liver and kidneys. Its primary function in the body is to transport fatty acids across cell membranes so that they can be metabolized in the mitochondria. Carnitine is used medicinally in the treatment of conditions such as Alzheimer's disease and is also a popular weight loss supplement. Some endurance athletes use it in the belief that it increases the body's fat-burning efficiency during exercise.

Unfortunately, studies have repeatedly shown that carnitine supplementation has no effect on fat utilization either at rest or during exercise and no effect on endurance performance. While carnitine is essential for fat utilization during exercise, it appears that athletes get as much as they need in the diet and that supplementation offers no additional benefit.

Carnitine supplementation is safe, if useless from the perspective of running performance. The typical dosage is 1 to 2 grams. Carnitine supplements are available in both pill and liquid forms.

COENZYME Q10 (CoQ10)

Enzymes are chemical compounds that facilitate vital chemical reactions in the body. Coenzymes, as their name suggests, are chemical compounds that play a secondary role in facilitating vital chemical reactions. CoQ10 is a coenzyme that is found naturally in a variety of foods, is also synthesized by the body and is present in its every cell. It aids in aerobic metabolism by transporting electrons within the mitochondria of muscle cells.

Because CoQ10 serves this function, and because CoQ10 is available only in small amounts in the diet, some scientists have reasoned that CoQ10 supplementation might enhance aerobic performance. But most studies have found that CoQ10 has no ergogenic effect. Supplementation only seems to be beneficial in those with CoQ10 deficiencies (a side effect of some cholesterol medications) and in those with heart conditions that limit the flow of oxygen to the heart (congestive heart failure, angina, and irregular heartbeat).

CoQ10 is also a powerful antioxidant. It has exhibited a remarkable capacity to limit oxidative tissue damage in patients with conditions ranging from Parkinson's disease to liver transplantation. However, it does not appear to have much effect on damage to muscle cells caused by oxygen radicals during exercise.

Doses of CoQ10 as high as 2,400 milligrams per day have been proven safe. There is no official recommended dosage of CoQ10, but individuals without significant health problems are generally advised not to take more than 100 milligrams daily. Consult your physician before taking a CoQ10 supplement for any medical reason.

CREATINE

Creatine has a stronger beneficial impact on athletic performance than any other safe and legal dietary supplement. The only problem is that, while it does wonderful things for strength, sprint, and power athletes, it has no proven beneficial effect on distance running performance. Nevertheless, it may still be worth taking.

The most common supplement form of creatine is creatine monohydrate. This compound is a precursor to a slightly different compound called creatine phosphate, which occurs naturally in the body and is one of the most important sources of energy for high-intensity (anaerobic) muscle contractions. Creatine phosphate provides energy so rapidly that it is the muscles' primary energy source for maximum-intensity efforts such as heavy weightlifting and sprinting. The muscles store it in extremely small amounts, though, so it lasts no longer than 15 seconds. This is one of the reasons you can't maintain a full sprint much longer than 15 seconds.

A tiny percentage of our creatine phosphate stores are synthesized in the body. The rest comes ready-made in protein-rich foods including fish and beef. But even these foods contain only very small amounts of creatine phosphate. That's why scientists in the 1990s began to look at creatine supplementation as a potential means to enhance high-intensity muscle performance (strength, speed, and power) by increasing the availability of this particular energy source in the muscles. Creatine monohydrate is readily converted to creatine phosphate in the body and it's relatively cheap to produce, so it quickly became the preferred supplement form of creatine.

As few as 5 days of creatine monohydrate supplementation increases creatine phosphate levels in the body by 10 to 40 percent. Dozens of research studies have shown that these increases translate directly into better athletic performance in a variety of anaerobic modalities. According to a comprehensive review of creatine studies by researchers at Baylor University, short-term creatine supplementation has been reported to improve maximal power and strength by 5 to 15 percent. It increases the amount of work performed during multiple sets of maximal-effort weight lifting by the same amount. It increases performance in a single sprint by 1 to 5 percent, and in multiple sprints by 5 to 15 percent. Moreover, when daily creatine supplementation is combined with appropriate training over a period of weeks, fitness gains are significantly enhanced. In other words, the same workouts result in faster muscle growth, strength gains, and improvements in high-intensity performance when daily creatine supplementation is added.

The only proven side effects of creatine supplementation are water retention and muscle weight gain, which is only to be expected because increases in strength and gains in muscle mass go hand in hand. (While gaining muscle weight is not a problem for strength and power athletes, in distance runners it has a costly negative impact on running economy.) Even long-term creatine supplementation has not been linked to any negative health consequences. However, creatine supplementation is not effective for every athlete. Some just don't respond to it, and among those who do, some respond more than others.

Creatine does not affect performance in any type of exercise lasting longer than 90 seconds. Yet even distance runners do (or should do) a small amount of very high-speed running and high-intensity strength training. Since creatine clearly enhances performance in these types of

(continued on page 196)

A SUMMARY OF DIETARY SUPPLEMENTS FOR RUNNERS

	What is it supposed to do?	Does it really work?
Caffeine	Boost endurance performance	Yes
Carnitine	Increase fat burning efficiency	No
CoQ10	Boost aerobic metabolism by transporting electrons inside muscle cell mitochondria	Only in those with CoQ10 deficiencies (a side effect of some cholesterol medications) and in those with heart conditions that limit the flow of oxygen to the heart (congestive heart failure, angina, and irregular heart beat).
Creatine	Boost strength, speed, and power; reduce muscle damage	Yes
Glucosamine and Chondroitin	Protect and rebuild joint cartilage; reduce joint pain; improve joint function	Effective in arthritis sufferers; not adequately studied in runners
Ginseng	Delay central nervous system fatigue; reduce muscle damage and inflammation	Existing research contradictory; more research required
Glutamine	Limits exercise induced immunosuppression; helps prevent overtraining syndrome; promotes muscle recovery	Yes
MSM	Reduce joint pain and inflammation; promote cartilage formation	More research is required

Is it safe?	What's the proper dosage?
Side effects include jitters and tension; insomnia, especially at higher doses; some habitual users become caffeine-dependent; it is not recommended for those with heart disease or high blood pressure	2–6 g/lb 1 hour before exercise
Yes	Standard dosage is 1–2 g/day
Yes	100 mg per day
Yes	20 g/day during 4-day loading phase then 2.5–5g/day
Yes	Typical dosages in studies are 1500 mg glucosamine and 800 mg chondroitin/day
Yes	Standard dosage amounts are usually in the range of 1–2 g/day
Yes	1–4 g/day is optimal; the best sources of supplemental glutamine are performance recovery drinks such as Endurox R4
Yes	Common dosage is 2–4 g/day

(CONTINUED ON NEXT PAGE)

A SUMMARY OF DIETARY SUPPLEMENTS FOR RUNNERS (CONTINUED)

	What is it supposed to do?	Does it really work?
Omega-3 Fatty Acids	Enhance blood oxygen transport; reduce post-exercise muscle inflammation	Study results have been generally negative, but supplementation is still recommended for general health
Sodium Citrate	Helps prevent muscular acidosis; boosts performance in races of 2– 15 minutes	Evidence is contradictory
Sodium Phosphate	Helps prevent muscular acidosis; improves blood oxygen transport	Early studies were promising, but more research is needed
Vitamins C and E	Reduce running-induced muscle damage and inflammation	Evidence is mostly supportive for vitamin E, mixed for vitamin C

training, it could indirectly enhance your race performances by boosting the fitness gains you derive from running short intervals and lifting weights—theoretically—as long as it doesn't cause you to gain too much muscle weight!

Another, completely different and highly intriguing benefit of creatine supplementation for distance runners was identified recently. New evidence suggests that creatine supplementation may reduce muscle damage during endurance exercise and thereby facilitate recovery. In a Brazilian study, runners who took supplemental creatine for 5 days before running a marathon exhibited less muscle soreness and inflammation afterward than runners who took a placebo.

I myself take supplemental creatine. My experience is that it does

Is it safe?	What's the proper dosage?
Yes	Recommended dosage for supplemental omega-3 is 1,000 mg/day; ratio of supplemental omega-3 to omega-6 should be at least 2:1
May cause gastrointestinal distress during running	Take 0.5 g/kg of body weight dissolved into a liter of flavored water 90 minutes before racing
Exceeding the recommended dosage may cause GI distress; long-term excessive intake may impair calcium balance	Take 1 g 4 times per day for 6 days preceding a race between 1 mile and 10K
Yes	Common dosages in studies showing benefits are in the range of 800–1,500 mg of vitamin C and 800–1,200 IU of vitamin E

indeed enhance the strength and power gains I get from lifting weights and doing plyometrics (jumping drills). Some runners complain that creatine supplementation causes them to gain more muscle weight than they can tolerate, but it has not done so in my case, perhaps because I maintain a high overall training volume. But it's possible that you would get very different results. In any case, because it has no other side effects, it can't hurt to try creatine supplementation if you're interested. On the other hand, even in the best case it's doubtful that creatine supplementation will give you more than a 1-percent performance boost, and that boost won't come cheaply. A 200-serving canister of unflavored creatine monohydrate powder (the most economical type of creatine supplement) costs about $40.

It's recommended that you begin supplementation with a 4- to 7-day loading period during which you take 20 grams per day (four doses of 5 grams each). Afterward, take 2.5 to 5 grams per day. Because insulin is needed to drive creatine into the muscle cells, you should mix the powder into fruit juice (or take the pills with fruit juice). Otherwise, you can buy the supplement as a flavored drink mix.

GLUCOSAMINE AND CHONDROITIN

Glucosamine and chondroitin are natural compounds found in joint cartilage. They have become popular as dietary supplements (usually in the form of glucosamine hydrochloride and chondroitin sulfate) among arthritis sufferers, athletes, and others experiencing joint pain and dysfunction. There is solid evidence that glucosamine and chondroitin supplements are effective in treating these symptoms and signs of cartilage damage or degeneration.

Joint cartilage connects bone to bone and helps absorb shock and control joint movements. Cartilage is made of thick bands of collagen woven together on a tissue framework of glycosaminoglycans (GAGs). Glucosamine is the major precursor to GAGs. Formation of GAGs is limited by the availability of glucosamine, which is made from glucose and glutamine in the body. Under normal circumstances plenty of glucosamine is available, but when GAGs are damaged through injury or arthritis, there may not be enough glucosamine available. This is when a glucosamine supplement might help.

Chondroitin, meanwhile, is the most abundant type of GAG. It is believed to play an important role in lubricating cartilage, as well as in stimulating the production of collagen, inhibiting inflammation, and counteracting certain enzymes responsible for breaking down cartilage.

Recently some well-designed studies have shown that, both individually and in combination, glucosamine hydrochloride and chondroitin sulfate supplements are effective in reducing joint pain associated with damaged cartilage, improving mobility in the affected joint, and limiting further cartilage deterioration. Almost all of these studies have involved patients with osteoarthritis, not runners or other athletes with joint pain caused by activity. While many runners believe that training causes a progressive wearing down of the knee cartilage that could eventually lead to osteoarthritis, the reality is that older runners are *less* likely to suffer from this condition than their sedentary counterparts.

Nevertheless, running often does inflame and damage cartilage in the knees and, to a lesser extent, the hips. Knee pain is the most common overuse injury among runners. Such pain does not always involve cartilage tissue, but in many cases it does. Can a glucosamine-chondroitin supplement prevent or effectively treat knee pain in runners? The short answer is, I don't know—nor does anyone else, because this question has not yet been formally studied. Most experts believe that glucosamine-chondroitin supplementation will eventually be proven to have some benefit in this regard. However, to expect a glucosamine-chondroitin supplement to prevent or completely heal full-blown knee injuries is like expecting a vitamin E supplement to prevent or heal skin damage caused by lying naked in the sun all day every day with no sunscreen. In other words, a glucosamine-chondroitin supplement does not address the root causes of cartilage damage in runners, which include poor stride mechanics and muscular imbalances. These problems must be corrected with strength exercises and stride modifications.

There are no official recommended doses of glucosamine and chondroitin. The average dose used in studies that have found a positive effect and no significant side effects is 1,500 milligrams per day of glucosamine and 800 milligrams per day of chondroitin. There is a wide disparity in the quality (i.e., purity) of various brands of these supplements, so ask a naturopathic doctor or a knowledge-able salesperson for recommendations before you buy, or consult www.consumerlab.com (as recommended previously).

GINSENG

Ginseng is an herb of Chinese origin that has been used medicinally for thousands of years. It has a variety of effects in the body, including antioxidant and anti-inflammatory influences and immune system balancing. It has been used successfully to prevent the development of cancerous tumors and to treat lung infection in patients with cystic fibrosis.

The effects of ginseng on exercise performance and post-exercise recovery are less clear and require further study. A recent Korean study found that supplementation with red ginseng (one of several ginseng varieties) increased endurance in rats by slowing the buildup of the hormone serotonin in the brain during exercise. Other studies, involving human subjects, have shown no ergogenic effect of ginseng during exercise.

Recent studies of the effects of ginseng on post-exercise recovery have produced promising results. Spanish researchers found that ginseng supplementation reduced muscle damage and inflammation in rats following exercise. But again, other research investigating different aspects of recovery in human subjects has shown no benefit of ginseng supplementation.

These contradictory results may be explained in part by the fact that various studies have used different ginseng species and a range of concentrations of the active ingredient. We're probably still years away from fully understanding whether, how, and to what degree ginseng supplementation may help runners and other athletes. In the meantime, we do know that long-term ginseng supplementation is considered safe, so if you want to experiment with it, feel free. The standard dose is usually in the range of 1 to 2 grams per day.

GLUTAMINE

Glutamine is classified as a conditionally essential amino acid. This means that, although your body can manufacture glutamine, there are circumstances in which it can't make glutamine fast enough to meet an increased demand for it. One of those times is following exercise.

As described in Chapter 1, glutamine is used at a very high rate during exercise. It is sent from the muscles to the liver and converted to glucose, which is then sent back to the muscles to provide energy. Plasma glutamine levels drop dramatically (45 percent in one study) during prolonged exercise and remain low for some time afterward. This leaves the body more susceptible to bacterial and viral infections, because glutamine is an important fuel for the immune system. Several studies have shown that taking supplemental glutamine after exercise lessens exercise-induced immunosuppression and reduces the risk of infection.

During periods of heavy training, many athletes become chronically glutamine-deficient. In one study, it was found that athletes had not recovered normal glutamine levels even 6 days after ceasing heavy training. Very low glutamine levels are almost invariably seen in athletes suffering from overtraining syndrome. This indicates that athletes in heavy training are unable to get enough glutamine in their diet to supplement what their bodies produce. This is not surprising, since glutamine comprises only about 5 percent of most dietary proteins, and most of the glutamine consumed in dietary proteins is used by the gut and never reaches the blood and muscles.

Taking supplemental glutamine is therefore a good idea for most runners and necessary for runners in heavy training. Perhaps the best way to get supplemental glutamine is in a recovery drink. Because glutamine also facilitates post-workout recovery by promoting protein synthesis and liver glycogen replenishment, it makes sense to get your supplemental glutamine from the same source that provides the other nutrients you need to optimize these components of recovery.

Most recovery drinks are made with whey protein, which has a high glutamine content, and a growing number of products are adding supplemental free glutamine. Choose a drink that contains at least 500 milligrams of glutamine, and preferably 1 gram or more. Some recovery drinks contain as many as 6 grams of glutamine per serving. That may be more than you need, but it's still safe. Oral doses of glutamine as high as 0.3 gram per kilogram of body weight have been administered without any signs of toxicity. Note that glutamine is easily derived from the branched-chain amino acids (leucine, isoleucine, and valine), which are also ingredients in some recovery drinks.

MSM

Methylsulfonylmethane (MSM) is a natural source of the essential mineral sulfur and is found in a variety of foods, including many fruits, vegetables, and grains, as well as dairy products. MSM is believed to reduce inflammation and its associated pain and to assist in the formation of joint cartilage. Supplemental MSM is therefore very popular among those with arthritis and is also gaining popularity among athletes for the treatment of muscle soreness. There is a lot of hype about MSM and a great deal of anecdotal evidence of its effectiveness, but as yet there is very little scientific proof. However, since it is completely nontoxic, it might be worth a try if you're looking for an alternative to aspirin or other anti-inflammatory medications. The typical dose is 2 to 4 grams per day.

OMEGA-3 FATTY ACIDS

Omega-3 fatty acids are a type of essential fat, meaning they cannot be synthesized in the body and must be obtained in adequate amounts in the diet. This is easier said than done, because omega-3 fatty acids are destroyed when the oils that contain them are processed or heated, and most of the omega-3 sources in the modern diet are processed and/or heated. Experts believe that omega-3 deficiency is one of the most widespread nutrient deficiencies in our society.

Omega-3 essential fatty acids create healthier cell membranes. In addition, they are important precursors to anti-inflammatory components of the immune system. Both of these effects are potentially valuable to runners. It has been suggested that by increasing the fluidity and deformability of red blood cells, EFA supplementation might enhance the ability of red blood cells to transport oxygen to the muscles. There has also been hope that EFA supplementation might reduce the inflammatory response after exercise and thereby reduce secondary muscle damage and delayed-onset muscle soreness.

Research, however, has not been kind to these hopes. In one study, a group of 20 runners received either a daily fish oil supplement (fish oil is high in omega-3s) or a placebo for 6 weeks prior to running a marathon. While fish oil supplementation did alter the composition of cell membranes, there was no effect on markers of muscle tissue inflammation after the marathon. Other studies have shown no effect of omega-3 supplementation on delayed-onset muscle soreness. And the hope that omega-3 supplementation might improve aerobic capacity has likewise not been borne out.

Does this mean that omega-3 supplementation is useless for runners? While it may be useless from a pure performance perspective, from the perspective of all-around health it appears to be quite beneficial. Omega-3 supplementation has been shown to improve cardiovascular health, sympathetic nervous system functioning, immune function, and skin health. For this reason, and because it is very difficult to get enough omega-3s from regular foods, omega-3 supplementation is advisable for everyone.

The American Heart Association recommends a daily omega-3 intake of 1,000 milligrams per day. Intake levels above 3,000 milligrams per day may be unhealthy. The most popular omega-3 supplements are fish oil, flaxseed oil, and various oil blends such as Udo's Choice. They are available in liquid and capsule form. Most omega-3 supplements are formulated to provide 500 to 1,000 milligrams per serving. Avoid oil supplements that contain omega-3 and omega-6 fatty acids in a ratio of less than 2:1, as omega-6 fatty acids are much easier to come by in the diet and research has shown that the benefits of getting more omega-3s are nullified when you increase your omega-6 intake disproportionately.

SODIUM CITRATE

Sodium citrate is a salt associated with citric acid. It occurs naturally in a variety of foods, including many fruits. It is also an intermediate product of aerobic metabolism in the human body. When consumed in food or produced in the body, sodium citrate quickly degrades into sodium bicarbonate (yes, baking soda), which functions as an acid buffer. In other words, it helps prevent body tissues from becoming too acidic.

It is believed that muscle tissue tends to become more acidic during high-intensity exercise (a phenomenon known as muscular acidosis). This tendency is caused by the leakage of loose protons and potassium ions from the muscle cells. Sodium bicarbonate, lactate, and other natural buffers neutralize these protons and ions and help prevent acidosis from getting out of hand. When acidosis does get out of hand, the electrical signals that cause your muscle fibers to contract (and relax) become interrupted and you experience fatigue.

There is some evidence that taking sodium citrate as a dietary supplement before high-intensity exercise delays fatigue by increasing the availability of sodium bicarbonate in the muscles. In slightly more than half of the tests performed, a benefit has been observed. In these studies, there is usually a wide range of responses. Some subjects get a big boost, others a small boost, and others none at all. Sodium citrate is believed to have no effect on performance in events lasting less than 2 minutes or longer than 15 minutes, where acidosis is not a major cause of fatigue, although a couple of studies have recorded a benefit in time trials lasting as long as 30 minutes.

The most reliable results seem to follow when about 0.5 gram of sodium citrate per kilogram of body weight is dissolved into a liter of flavored water (it's unpalatable in plain water) and consumed about 90 minutes before racing. Note that large amounts of sodium citrate— and this dosage most certainly qualifies as a large amount—cause gastrointestinal distress in some people. For this reason, and because some people do not respond to sodium citrate even when they can tolerate it, test it in a workout context once or twice before you begin using it in race situations.

SODIUM PHOSPHATE

Phosphate is a nonmetallic element and the second most abundant mineral in the human body, after calcium. It combines with various other minerals in the body to serve a wide range of functions. Sodium phosphate is mainly responsible for regulating acid-base balance in body tissues. It is also a major component of a compound that helps release oxygen from red blood cells.

Scientists believe that, like sodium citrate, sodium phosphate plays a role in preventing muscular acidosis during very intense exercise. For many years, researchers have speculated that taking supplemental sodium phosphate, or "phosphate loading," prior to shorter races might increase sodium phosphate stores in the body and thereby enhance its ability to prevent muscular acidosis and to release oxygen from red blood cells, thereby boosting performance.

A pair of well-designed studies conducted in the late 1980s and early 1990s found that VO_2max and lactate thresholds were increased in runners following a 6-day phosphate-loading protocol. One would have expected the promising results of these studies to inspire both follow-up studies and widespread interest in phosphate loading, but they have not, for whatever reason. A later review provided further validation of these results.

It's impossible to wholeheartedly recommend phosphate loading based on the results of only two studies and one review. However, I can say that it *probably* is effective, and it's also perfectly safe, so there's no reason not to try it. The loading protocol used with success in the studies mentioned consisted of taking 1 gram of sodium phosphate 4 times per day for 6 days. There are potential side effects of exceeding this dosage, namely, nausea, stomach cramps, and diarrhea. Long-term excessive phosphate intake can leech calcium from bones.

Note that phosphate loading is unlikely to be beneficial prior to races longer than 8K to 10K, as muscular acidosis is not a factor in such events.

VITAMINS C AND E

Vitamins C and E have a long list of functions in every person, but in runners these vitamins have a special, extra function, which is to reduce muscle damage caused by oxygen radicals and other free radicals during and after workouts and races. A number of studies have shown that runners (and other athletes) experience less muscle damage when they take vitamin C and vitamin E supplements either separately or in tandem.

In a Japanese study, a group of runners was divided into two subgroups, one of which received a daily vitamin E supplement, the other a placebo. After 4 weeks, both groups were subjected to 6 days of unusually hard training. Researchers then measured the amount of muscle damage in the runners and found it was much lower in the vitamin E group than in the placebo group.

Similarly, a South African study looked at the effects of short-term vitamin C supplementation on anti-inflammatory hormones and proteins following the 90K Comrades Marathon (an ultramarathon). For 7 days preceding the race, runners received either 1,500 milligrams of vitamin C, 500 milligrams of vitamin C, or a placebo. The runners receiving the larger dose of vitamin C exhibited significantly lower levels of adrenaline and anti-inflammatory polypeptides after the race than members of the other two groups. The researchers took this as an indirect indication that they had experienced less muscle damage during the grueling race.

Other studies have investigated the combined effect of vitamin C and vitamin E supplementation. An Oregon State University study measured lipid peroxidation in supplemented and nonsupplemented runners after a 50K ultramarathon. Lipid peroxidation is damage to cell membranes caused by free radicals. In this study, combined vitamin C and E supplementation showed a strong protective effect against such damage.

It makes sense to take supplemental vitamin C and vitamin E together, because they work synergistically. Vitamin C helps to replenish your body's vitamin E supply. The doses used in the above-mentioned studies and in other studies showing benefits are in the range of 800 to 1,500 milligrams of vitamin C and 800 to 1,200 IU of vitamin E daily. These doses are safe and found in many individual vitamin and multivitamin supplements. Some recovery drinks also contain vitamins C and E in fairly large amounts. I recommend that you get your supplemental vitamin C and vitamin E from *either* a tablet *or* a recovery drink (if you use a drink such as Ultragen that contains them in tablet-level amounts), not from both, because it is possible to get too much of these good things.

A recent scientific review found that long-term consumption of more than 400 IU of vitamin E daily slightly increases all-cause death risk. However, this effect may be relevant only to patients who already have a degenerative disease, as none of the studies reviewed had examined healthy subjects. Further research is needed to determine a safe maximum vitamin E dosage for healthy individuals. In the meantime, you may wish to pursue a cautious middle ground and limit your supplemental intake to no more than 400 IU daily.

CHAPTER 10

RUNNERS WITH SPECIAL NUTRITION NEEDS

Pursuing optimal performance nutrition is like running a road race. Some runners start at the front, others in the middle, and still others at the back. Some begin with a lot of experience under their belt, while others start as beginners. And individual runners compete in various categories sorted by age, gender, and sometimes even size. But everyone moves toward the same finish line. Individual runners begin their pursuit of optimal performance nutrition in different places and as representatives of various groups. Your path toward this destination may look a little different from the paths of other runners based on your age, gender, size, preferences, special needs, and other factors. But the final destination for every runner is a set of nutrition habits that maximizes overall health and running performance.

In an earlier chapter, I discussed the basic nutritional needs that are universal throughout the human race. These include the need for variety in the diet and the need to balance energy intake with energy use. In addition, I alluded to the existence of individual needs based on genetic differences. There are also nutritional needs and challenges that are neither universal nor individual but specific to certain groups of people. One obvious example of such a group is vegetarians, who must meet their nutritional needs in different ways than those who eat animal foods.

A sizeable number of the nutrition questions I receive from runners come from representatives of one or another subgroup that has some special nutritional needs or challenges. The most commonly represented subgroups are youth runners (these questions usually come from parents), women runners, older runners, overweight runners, diabetic runners, and vegetarian runners. In this chapter, I will address some of the questions that I am asked most often by members of each of these groups.

YOUTH RUNNERS

As a parent, one of the best things you can do for your child is to pass along your passion for running. While you're at it, be sure to pass along the secrets to performance nutrition as well.

Q: How are my child's everyday nutritional needs different from mine?

A: After infancy, the everyday nutritional needs of children are similar to those of adults, but not identical. Growth is the primary factor that makes the general nutritional needs of youth runners somewhat different from those of adults. Normal growth is encoded in the genetic material of each person, but this plan cannot be realized without appropriate nutrition.

In our society, most children have no difficulty consuming enough calories to fuel normal growth. In fact, the real problem is not undernourishment but overnourishment, resulting in overweight and obesity. Currently, a third of American children are overweight. One of the primary causes of this alarming problem is inactivity. If your child is a recreational or competitive runner, she's already doing the best thing she can do to avoid becoming overweight. The single greatest risk factor for childhood obesity is obese parents, so perhaps the most effective thing *you* can do to raise normal-weight children is to maintain a healthy weight yourself.

Beyond protein and total energy, other nutrients that are especially vital for childhood growth are iodide, zinc, iron, and vitamins A, B_2 (riboflavin), C, and D. Iodide is most abundant in sea salt, iodized salt, and seafood. Vitamin A, riboflavin, and zinc are easily found in a wide range of animal foods (including seafood) and vegetables. Vitamin D is most abundant in dairy foods and seafood, vitamin C in a long list of fruits and vegetables, and iron in animal foods.

Q: What can I do to ensure my child eats right?

A: Children depend on their parents to shape their diet and optimize their nourishment. This awesome responsibility is enough to make many parents reach for the panic button, but it need not. Here are four simple rules you can follow to nourish your child well without driving yourself nuts in the process.

Lead by example. Children do as their parents do more than they do as their parents say. In other words, they naturally take after their parents in a majority of their lifestyle habits, regardless of whether their parents overtly encourage or discourage any specific habit. If you exercise regularly and enjoy it, your children probably will too, without your having to command it. On the other hand, if you smoke cigarettes, your children will most likely follow your lead, no matter how much you discourage them.

So if you want your children to maintain a wholesome, well-balanced diet, do so yourself. This goes beyond simply serving your children the same healthy meals you eat. Show your enthusiasm for healthy food and avoid nagging your child about food choices, especially if you're not making the same choices for yourself.

Give them lessons. As you learn about nutrition, share some of this knowledge with your child. This will empower him to make good nutrition choices throughout life. Don't go about it pedantically, but casually, for example by naming one or two key nutrients that are in the foods you're eating for tonight's dinner, and what these nutrients do for your child's body. Personalize the lesson. Kids are intensely curious about most everything, but you have to take the right approach or they'll tune you out.

Work with your child's tastes. Many children are picky eaters. Most of them grow out of it. Few can be forced out of it, so be patient and do your best to feed your child nutritious foods that she enjoys, without overindulging her pickiness if it's extreme. It's okay and even important to challenge your child to expand her tastes, but you have to choose your battles.

Avoid using less nutritious foods as rewards for eating healthy ones. ("Finish your Brussels sprouts and you can have a hot fudge sundae.") This only reinforces the value system that underlies fussy tastes. It's better to offer nonfood rewards. ("Finish your Brussels sprouts and I'll take you swimming tomorrow afternoon.")

Don't go overboard. As important as raising your child on healthy foods is raising your child to have a healthy attitude toward food. A healthy attitude toward food is one whereby eating healthily is a pleasure and not an obsession or worry. In coaching your child to eat well, avoid making the rules too rigid, overemphasizing the negative aspects of unhealthy eating, and making too big a fuss about the whole thing.

These days, I see too many parents who are afraid to ever feed their children the wrong thing, and as a result they're raising children who are afraid of food. Relax! It's not that serious. There's no such thing as a perfect diet, but there is most certainly such a thing as a diet that's good enough!

Q: What are my child's hydration and energy needs during running?

A: During exercise, youth runners should do exactly as adult runners do: drink a quality sports drink (or energy gels plus water) every 10 to 12 minutes throughout all workouts lasting longer than 45 minutes and throughout all high-intensity workouts. Youth runners get the same benefits from this practice as adult runners, which include greater endurance, better performance in high-intensity workouts, reduced muscle damage, and faster postrun recovery.

I regularly encounter parents who associate sugar with consequences such as obesity, hyperactivity, and diabetes, and who worry that the sugars in ergogenic aids might be harmful to their children. This worry, although understandable, is without foundation as long as sports drinks and energy gels are used specifically to fuel exercise. Ergogenic aids enhance running performance, and by doing this they enhance all of the benefits of running, among them improved body composition and greater insulin sensitivity. Neither children nor adults should make a habit of consuming sports drinks and energy gels outside of exercise. In this case, the sugars they contain will contribute to fat storage and related issues.

Q: Should I allow my child to use nutritional supplements?

A: According to recent surveys, use of dietary supplements (and performance-enhancing drugs) among college and high school athletes is on the rise. Results from the latest NCAA survey indicate that 42 percent of student-athletes use one or more types of supplements, and of these, 62 percent began supplementing in high school. A survey of male high school athletes in Louisiana showed that nearly 50 percent had tried a supplement at least once.

What is most alarming about this situation is that many student-athletes are using supplements that are banned and/or carry significant health risks. It is clear that these individuals are poorly educated about the true effects of supplements and their status with respect to the rules of their sport. Not all supplements are illegal or dangerous, but proper education should precede the choice to use even those supplements that are benign and condoned by the International Olympic Committee, the NCAA, and state athletic associations. Few student-athletes are getting this education from their coaches, so it will probably have to come from you.

All of the nutritional supplements discussed in Chapter 9 of this book are safe for children. Nevertheless, if I were the parent of a young runner I would actively discourage my son or daughter from using most of them. The purpose of using a supplement such as ginseng or caffeine is to potentially provide a very slight performance edge after every other measure to enhance performance through training and nutrition has already been taken. In other words, supplements come last in a runner's performance regimen. Youth runners have so much opportunity to improve through normal development and training that using supplements is simply premature for them, and delivers the wrong message about the proper place of supplements in a runner's regimen. In allowing a child to use supplements too soon, I believe there is a risk of teaching a magic bullet mentality that could result in unhealthy choices later, such as the choice to take anabolic steroids or unsafe diet pills.

The one exception is supplemental omega-3 fatty acids, which I recommend for all children because they are necessary for optimal health. There are several omega-3 supplements formulated especially for children. Use them according to label directions.

WOMEN RUNNERS

The sport of running has grown tremendously in the last 20 years, and the primary factor driving this growth has been a sharp rise in the participation of women. Along with this explosion in participation has come a keen interest in issues specific to female runners, including nutrition.

Q: How do my general nutrition needs differ from those of a male runner?

A: Contrary to what many women have been led to believe, the nutritional needs of female runners are not significantly different from those of male runners. However, female runners often eat differently from male runners in ways that prevent them from meeting some of their nutritional needs.

For example, many women believe that they require more calcium than males. They do not. The reason some women believe their calcium needs are higher is that women are more likely than men to develop osteoporosis (dangerously low bone density), and calcium is the main mineral ingredient of bone tissue. The problem of osteoporosis is so widespread that doctors and nutrition experts are constantly urging women to consume more calcium. But the calcium deficiency that sometimes contributes to osteoporosis is not due to higher calcium needs; rather, it is due to lower average calcium consumption in women.

A lot of women avoid calcium-rich dairy foods in an effort to avoid fat. This point leads us to the core nutritional challenge that female runners (and women in general) face as a group: social pressure to be thin. As we all know, in our culture there is a double standard that makes fuller body shapes less acceptable in women than in men. This standard motivates millions of women—and girls—to undernourish themselves in a misguided effort to look the way they think they're supposed to look.

Athletes, including runners, are as likely to be affected as nonathletes. In fact, compulsive exercise is another unhealthy way that some females attempt to achieve a warped ideal of thinness. While a great number of female runners do develop serious eating disorders such as anorexia nervosa, much greater numbers undernourish themselves to a milder (but still unhealthy) degree. This broader phenomenon is often referred to as disordered eating. (Eating disorders are specific and severe forms of disordered eating.)

The marketing of special vitamins, energy bars, and other foods and supplements for women gives the impression that, when it comes to nutrition, "men are from Mars and women are from Venus." In addition, research studies showing special benefits of specific nutrients for women (for example, studies show omega-3 fatty acids reduce the risk of breast cancer) are often misinterpreted as evidence that these nutrients are especially important for women. But the actual differences between male and female nutrition needs are very slight. Because our bodies are different, we use the same nutrients somewhat differently, but we need essentially the same nutrients.

The real issue is that women are more likely than men to fail to meet the nutritional needs that are common to both genders. Focus on eating the way a human being should instead of the way you may have been led to believe a woman should.

Q: What is the nutrition-related condition called the "triad" that affects female runners and how do I avoid it?

A: The female athlete triad is a disturbingly common condition in female athletes. As its name suggests, it is made up of three health conditions that have a dietary link: disordered eating, amenorrhea (cessation of monthly periods), and osteoporosis. Often, but not always, these conditions are present simultaneously in female athletes who are undernourishing their bodies due to negative body image. Two-thirds of American women report being dissatisfied with their body weight.

Disordered eating is typically the trigger of the triad. Inadequate energy intake combined with intense training can cause a woman's body fat level to fall so low that the ovaries no longer produce enough estrogen. This hormone is critical for normal periods and also for bone formation. Calcium deficiency, when combined with low estrogen, makes the bones even thinner and more brittle, thereby increasing the risk of stress fractures.

Here are some tips for women runners to achieve adequate nutrition:

Don't eat by your own rules. Eat by the established rules as explained in this book and other credible resources. And don't make up your own ideal body weight. Your ideal body weight is whatever body weight you end up with after consistently eating right and training well for several months. Focus on the process, not arbitrary goals that may or may not be realistic.

The difficulty is that individuals with eating disorders are as likely to have an unrealistic sense of what they are actually eating as they are to have a warped body image. Therefore, it's a good idea to conduct a reality check by keeping a food journal for a few days and using a food count guide to tally the number of calories you are consuming. Compare this figure against the recommended daily caloric intake for a woman of your age, weight, and activity level. (You can find simple daily calorie requirement calculators on various Web sites, such as www.changingshape.com.) These numbers should be nearly equal (allowing for the approximate nature of calorie counting and daily requirement calculators). If you are surprised to find your intake too low, you should meet with a registered dietitian to discuss your diet and explore the possibility that your eating is disordered.

Another way to keep your beliefs about your eating habits in touch with reality is to monitor your running performance. If you are consistently undereating, your running performance will eventually begin to worsen. A drop in running performance that does not have any other obvious explanation (e.g., you took 2 weeks off) should raise a red flag suggesting the possibility that your eating is disordered.

Consider your body image, not your body weight. If you are not satisfied with your body weight, yet your body composition is in the healthy range (see page 77), the real problem may be your body image. Talk to your doctor about it.

Beware of restricting certain types of foods. Many female athletes eliminate dairy from their diet or become vegetarians to facilitate weight loss. What they really end up doing is undernourishing themselves— eating too few calories, or not getting enough of specific nutrients that are most abundant in animal foods (e.g., protein, calcium, and iron). There is really no legitimate health reason to avoid dairy foods or meat. So unless you have an ethical or religious reason for doing so, I don't recommend it.

See a doctor if . . . you miss three periods not due to pregnancy, or if you suffer frequent stress fractures.

OLDER RUNNERS

The percentage of runners over age 45 has increased by more than 30 percent in the last 5 years. This is due in part to the fact that the sport's retention rate is growing: the number of people who have been running for 10 years or more has also increased substantially in recent years. Nutrition is critical to running well over the long haul.

Q: How do my nutritional needs change as I get older?

A: Like youth runners and women runners, older runners do not have nutritional needs that are substantially different from those of runners in general. What is different about older runners, however, is that they can't get away with not eating properly the way a younger person might. In other words, the nutrition guidelines that are important for younger runners are even more important for older runners.

This is especially true for recovery nutrition. Older runners are more susceptible to muscle damage caused by eccentric muscle contractions (muscle contractions wherein the muscle lengthens as it contracts) and are not able to repair this damage as quickly between workouts. As I mentioned in earlier chapters, you can reduce muscle damage during running by drinking a sports drink containing carbohydrate and amino acids or protein. You can also greatly accelerate muscle tissue repair by consuming these same nutrients within 45 minutes of completing a run. But whereas a 20-year-old runner might be able to stray from these guidelines somewhat without noticeable consequences, a 50-year-old runner will almost certainly compromise his or her recovery severely.

Nutrition habits play an important role in maintaining muscle mass and strength. The older a runner gets, the less he can take his nutrition habits for granted in this regard. After age 35, we tend to gradually lose muscle mass, mainly because we produce smaller amounts of anabolic hormones such as growth hormone. Adequate protein intake is essential for muscle maintenance. Research has also shown that athletes who practice correct recovery nutrition habits are better able to maintain muscle mass.

Proper nutrition alone is not enough. Unless you combine adequate protein intake with exercise, you will not succeed in slowing aging-related muscle atrophy. Running is exercise, of course, and running has been shown to delay and slow muscle loss in older runners. But to really do the job properly you must supplement your running with strength training. Again, younger runners can likely avoid strength training and not lose muscle mass. (For injury prevention, strength training will benefit you no matter what your age.) But once you pass age 35, strength training becomes truly indispensable for maintaining muscle mass—along with adequate protein intake and correct post-workout nutrition habits.

Our daily energy needs also tend to decrease gradually as we age. This is primarily an effect of a simultaneous decrease in the resting metabolic rate (RMR), which in turn is partly due to muscle loss. One reason most adults gain weight steadily throughout adulthood is that they continue to eat the same amount despite the fact that their RMR is going down. This phenomenon does not occur in runners and other endurance athletes, however. In a study at the University of Colorado, female runners and swimmers aged 50 to 72 had the same RMR as women aged 21 to 35, whereas the RMR of sedentary women aged 50 to 72 was 10 percent lower on average. So the bottom line is that if you stay in shape throughout your life, the amount you eat should not have to change.

DIABETIC RUNNERS

Diabetes is a disease that has important implications for how runners fuel themselves before, during, and after workouts. For the rest of us, what's at stake in eating and drinking properly at these times is mainly performance. For diabetic runners, health is at stake is well.

There are two forms of diabetes. Type 1 diabetes occurs when the body's own immune system attacks and destroys the cells that produce insulin in the pancreas. The inability of the pancreas to produce adequate amounts of insulin inhibits the delivery of glucose to cells throughout the body. This leads to a whole chain of problems that are common in those with type 1 diabetes, including fatigue, damage to the kidneys and eyes, and atherosclerosis. Type 1 diabetes is usually diagnosed in people under the age of 20. Regular monitoring of blood glucose levels, careful control of the diet, and insulin therapy are required to manage the condition.

Type 2 diabetes is more common and tends to develop later in life. It begins when body tissues become insulin resistant as an indirect effect of high levels of fat storage (more than 50 percent of type 2 diabetics are obese), resulting in a backlog of glucose in the blood that causes the pancreas to pump out even more insulin, but to no avail. After a while the pancreas can wear out and lose much of its capacity to produce insulin, compounding the problem. People with type 2 diabetes experience many of the same health problems as those with type 1. Insulin therapy is required only for people with type 2 diabetes who reach the point of pancreatic exhaustion. There are also some prescription drugs that are effective in controlling type 2 diabetes. Managing diabetes of both types is all about managing blood glucose levels. In addition to dietary control, glucose monitoring, medication, and insulin therapy, exercise is also an effective tool to keep blood glucose in the proper range, and it can even reverse type 2 diabetes to some degree.

Q: As a diabetic runner, what risks do I face? Can I still be a successful runner?

A: Many successful runners and even world-class athletes have diabetes. Nevertheless, there are special risks involved in exercising with diabetes, so serious runners who happen to be diabetic need to be careful in their approach to training. And you may find that the disease hinders your athletic performance somewhat (because the muscles can't get as much glucose to provide energy).

People with type 1 diabetes are prone to hypoglycemia (low blood glucose) during exercise. Even nondiabetic runners experience hypoglycemia sometimes during the later stages of marathons and especially long workouts, but diabetics may encounter it after just a few minutes of exercise, and it can be deadly. Symptoms of hypoglycemia include fatigue, light-headedness, dizziness, and disorientation. Exercise actually tends to mask the symptoms of hypoglycemia (compared to rest), so diabetic athletes often experience delayed-onset hypoglycemia after a workout. For this reason, it is critically important to check your glucose level after the workout and eat carbohydrate and/or take insulin accordingly. People with type 2 diabetes are less prone to hypoglycemia during exercise, but some drugs for type 2 diabetes increase the risk, so if you take one, check with your doctor about switching. Reducing your insulin dosage before running can help prevent hypoglycemia.

The opposite problem—hyperglycemia, or dangerously high blood glucose—is also a risk in runners with diabetes. While moderate exercise tends to lower the blood glucose level, very long or intense runs can trigger a stress response that increases it, and this is more likely to occur in those who have diabetes.

As a runner with diabetes you must learn how various types of workouts affect your blood glucose level, because there are significant individual differences in this regard. It is also important to train under the supervision of a physician. You should demonstrate a consistent ability to keep your blood glucose level under control before you embark upon a serious training program, and you should never begin a workout unless your blood glucose is at a safe level (3 to 10 mmol/L).

Q: How are my sports nutrition needs different from those of nondiabetic runners?

A: If you have diabetes, doctors recommend eating a healthy meal containing at least 50 percent low-glycemic carbohydrates within 2 hours before exercising. Hydrating throughout exercise is also important, not only for the usual reasons but also because it helps to normalize blood glucose.

Carbohydrate intake during running is likewise even more important for the diabetic runner than for other runners, to prevent hypoglycemia. Doctors recommend consumption of at least 40 grams of carbohydrate per hour. The best source of fluid and carbohydrate is a quality sports drink. Many people with diabetes believe they should not consume sports drinks because they are high in sugar, and doctors always advise them to steer clear of sugary foods in their everyday eating. But this prohibition does not hold during exercise, except for those who are prone to hyperglycemia during exercise.

OVERWEIGHT RUNNERS

Running is one of the best weight loss tools on earth. Millions of overweight men and women take up running primarily for the sake of losing weight. There's one simple question I hear over and over from these individuals.

Q: I run mainly for weight loss. Should I eat and run the same way thin runners do, or do I require a special program?

A: As I explained in Chapter 4, achieving your ideal body composition is a natural and inevitable by-product of training and eating for optimal running performance. In other words, you don't need to consciously try to lose a certain number of pounds or to achieve a certain goal weight. The only way to know how much you should weigh (and what is your ideal body fat percentage) is to eat right, train smart, and see where you end up. Put another way, if you put your running performance first, your weight and body composition will surely follow.

There is an exception to this guideline, however. Most overweight beginning runners who are not necessarily concerned about running performance should initially follow a short-term diet and exercise program that is focused entirely on weight (fat) loss. The reasons are mainly psychological. Maintaining motivation is paramount when you're beginning an exercise program or modifying your diet in pursuit of weight loss. As you probably know, most people abandon such initiatives within a few weeks or months, so any trick that can be used to increase adherence should be exploited.

In my experience, the following three strategies strongly increase motivation and adherence:

Set concrete, short-term weight loss goals. Looking ahead to a lifetime of eating right and exercising can be overwhelming when you're just getting started. Setting a short-term initial goal is a lot more manageable. I recommend setting a goal of losing 10 to 25 pounds in 12 weeks. Twelve weeks is long enough to achieve outstanding results, yet short enough to still seem manageable. Of course, the whole idea is that by the time those 12 weeks have passed, you will have come to enjoy eating right and exercising and adherence is no longer a concern.

As I mentioned in Chapter 4, losing weight is not exactly the point, because not all weight loss is good weight loss. But there's nothing wrong with setting a sensible weight loss goal, because for many people it is the most highly motivating type of goal to pursue. It is critical that your goal be sensible given your current weight, your likely ideal weight, your diet and exercise history, and perhaps other factors. Nobody should set a goal of losing more than 25 pounds in a 12-week period.

Follow a highly structured diet and exercise program. Most people prefer to follow a detailed weight loss program that tells them exactly what they should do. This allows them to relax mentally and put all of their energy into doing instead of having to divide their energy between doing and thinking.

Start slowly and progress gradually. Beginning a new exercise program and embarking upon a new way of eating are big changes. Doing too much too soon in either area can be overwhelming and may result in a quick burnout (or injury, in the case of running).

In his popular book *8 Weeks to Optimal Health,* alternative medicine guru Andrew Weil, MD, recommends an approach to building a healthier lifestyle whereby the "dieter" makes just one new dietary change per week, maintaining changes from the preceding weeks as the program moves along. After the full 8 weeks, the dieter has radically transformed his or her diet for the better, but in a subtle and gentle way. No wonder Weil's book was such a hit!

I recommend that you take a similar approach to realizing a short-term weight loss goal. Here are 12 dietary changes that can help you lose 10 to 25 pounds over a 12-week period.

Week 1: Substitute water for fruit juices and sodas.
Week 2: Substitute a whole grain staple for a refined grain staple (wheat bread instead of white bread, for example).
Week 3: Stop eating when your fullness level reaches 3 or 4 on a 1-to-5 scale.
Week 4: Substitute low-fat dairy products for whole milk dairy products.

(continued on page 228)

RUNNING FOR WEIGHT LOSS

Here's a 12-week beginner's running program that you can follow while you're progressing through the sequence of dietary changes on pages 225 and 228. It assumes you have not been running recently and therefore begins with walk-jog workouts to allow your legs to adapt to repetitive impact. Also in-

	Monday	Tuesday	Wednesday
Week 1	Off	Walk 30 minutes w/ 8 × 1-minute jog	Strength 20 minutes
Week 2	Off	Walk 35 minutes w/ 12 × 1-minute jog	Strength 20 minutes
Week 3	Off	Walk 40 minutes w/ 8 × 2½-minute jog	Strength 20 minutes
Week 4	Off	Walk 40 minutes w/ 10-minute jog	Strength 20 minutes
Week 5	Off	Run 20 minutes	Strength 20 minutes
Week 6	Off	Run 24 minutes	Strength 20 minutes
Week 7	Off	Run 26 minutes	Strength 20 minutes
Week 8	Off	Run 24 minutes	Strength 20 minutes
Week 9	Off	Run 30 minutes	Strength 20 minutes
Week 10	Off	Run 32 minutes	Strength 20 minutes
Week 11	Off	Run 35 minutes	Strength 20 minutes
Week 12	Off	Run 30 minutes	Strength 20 minutes

cluded is one weekly cross-training workout (choose any nonimpact cardio ac-tivity, such as swimming or bicycling). Cross-training will allow you to maximize weight loss while minimizing your risk of injury. Two weekly strength workouts are also included to promote injury prevention and muscular conditioning.

Thursday	Friday	Saturday	Sunday
Walk 30 minutes w/ 8 × 1-minute jog	Cross-train 30 minutes	Strength 20 minutes	Walk 40 minutes w/ 10 × 1-minute jog
Walk 35 minutes w/ 12 × 1-minute jog	Cross-train 30 minutes	Strength 20 minutes	Walk 40 minutes w/ 8 × 2-minute jog
Walk 40 minutes w/ 8 × 3-minute jog	Cross-train 35 minutes	Strength 20 minutes	Walk 40 minutes w/ 4 x 5-minute jog
Walk 40 minutes w/ 12-minute jog	Cross-train 30 minutes	Strength 20 minutes	Run 20 minutes
Run 20 minutes	Cross-train 40 minutes	Strength 20 minutes	Run 24 minutes
Run 24 minutes	Cross-train 45 minutes	Strength 20 minutes	Run 28 minutes
Run 26 minutes	Cross-train 45 minutes	Strength 20 minutes	Run 32 minutes
Run 24 minutes	Cross-train 40 minutes	Strength 20 minutes	Run 24 minutes
Run 30 minutes	Cross-train 45 minutes	Strength 20 minutes	Run 36 minutes
Run 32 minutes	Cross-train 45 minutes	Strength 20 minutes	Run 40 minutes
Run 35 minutes	Cross-train 45 minutes	Strength 20 minutes	Run 45 minutes
Run 30 minutes	Cross-train 45 minutes	Strength 20 minutes	Run 40 minutes

Week 5: Add one to two servings of vegetables to your daily diet.

Week 6: Reduce your consumption of fried foods to 1 to 2 servings per week.

Week 7: Add 1 to 2 daily servings of fresh fruits to your diet.

Week 8: Reduce your consumption of refined sugar, caffeine, and alcohol.

Week 9: Introduce healthy midmorning and midafternoon snacks.

Week 10: Introduce immediate post-workout "recovery" meals, snacks, or supplements.

Week 11: Eliminate eating in front of screens (TV and computer).

Week 12: Begin eating more slowly.

If any of these suggested changes does not apply to you (perhaps you don't drink alcohol or coffee), replace it with something similar in spirit. A good general guideline for dietary changes to facilitate weight loss is substituting something healthier for something less healthy (such as substituting old-fashioned oatmeal for doughnuts). Another good source of weekly changes is the larger goal of working your way toward eating 6 times a day. If you tend to skip breakfast, for example, start eating it every day beginning in Week 3, or Week 8, or whenever you need an alternative change.

By the time you reach the end of Week 12, you will have lost at least 10 pounds of excess fat, supposing you have at least 10 to lose. If this schedule of layered changes seems too subtle and gentle to achieve such a result, bear in mind, you'll be working out too!

VEGETARIAN RUNNERS

Just yesterday I received another e-mail message from a runner who was considering becoming a vegetarian. Here is the question she asked me, and an expanded version of my reply.

Q: I am thinking about switching to a vegetarian diet mainly for health reasons, but will it also help me run better?

A: A vegetarian diet is not necessarily healthier than a well-balanced omnivorous diet. You can optimize your nutrition with or without animal foods. You can also fail to optimize your nutrition with or without animal foods. Let your values and preferences determine whether you go vegetarian. Don't fool yourself into thinking it's a health-based decision.

There are several categories of vegetarianism. They include the following:

Lacto-Ovo Vegetarian. This diet includes eggs and dairy foods, but no meat. It is the least restrictive form of vegetarianism. There are also lacto vegetarians who eat dairy foods but not eggs.

Vegan. This diet excludes all animal foods including eggs, dairy foods, and fish. A distinction is sometimes made between vegans and pure vegetarians. Vegans eliminate not only foods that contain animal products, but also foods whose production involves animals in any way, even when these foods do not actually contain animal parts —a list that includes gelatin, honey, and refined sugar. Pure vegetarians allow themselves to eat such foods.

Fruitarian. This diet comprises nothing but fruits. While incredibly restrictive, it's not quite as restrictive as you might first think, because many foods that we consider vegetables, such as cucumbers and tomatoes, are technically fruits.

Macrobiotic. This is a vegetarian diet of Japanese origin that is based on the health principle of balance between yin ("female energy") and yang ("masculine energy"). In addition to excluding all animal foods, it excludes a variety of plant-based foods that are considered "too yin" (sugar, coffee, tropical fruits, etc.). It is also a strictly organic diet. The primary constituents of the macrobiotic diet are whole grains, fresh vegetables, beans, and soups and broths.

Raw. This diet comprises only raw plant foods, including soaked and sprouted grains.

Fruitarian, strict macrobiotic, and raw diets are, in my view, too restrictive to provide optimal nutrition, especially for athletes. Fruitarian diets are likely to be deficient in a long list of nutrients, including protein, iron, and zinc. Strict macrobiotic diets are known to be deficient in vitamins B_{12} and D, calcium, and iron. And raw diets are based on a misguided belief that cooking makes plant foods less nourishing. Often the opposite is true. Cooking broccoli, for example, breaks down some of its tough cellulose so that the vitamins, minerals, and phytonutrients it contains can be more readily absorbed.

If you're going to go vegetarian, I recommend that you do so as a lacto-ovo vegetarian, lacto vegetarian, pure vegetarian, or vegan. On any of these diets, I believe it is possible to obtain optimal performance nutrition.

As I first mentioned back in Chapter 2, the more variety you have in your diet, the easier it is to meet all of your nutrition needs. Vegetarianism is no exception to this rule. All forms of vegetarianism are defined by voluntary restrictions in the variety of foods consumed, which makes it somewhat more challenging to meet all of your nutritional needs. To achieve optimal performance nutrition as a vegetarian, you need to eat in a way that "makes up for" these restrictions.

The first concern for vegetarian runners is obtaining enough total energy (calories). The best way to make sure you're getting enough daily energy is to monitor your weight, body fat percentage, and running performance. A trend toward losing weight while maintaining or even increasing your body fat percentage indicates a chronic energy deficiency. An extremely low body fat percentage indicates the same. In terms of running performance, an unexpected stagnation or decline in fitness, slow recovery from workouts, and frequent injuries and illnesses are also common indicators of inadequate caloric intake.

As a vegetarian runner. you must also make sure your diet includes abundant plant (and supplemental) sources of the several nutrients that animal foods generally contain in the greatest amounts: specifically, protein, calcium, iron, and vitamins B_2 and B_{12}. Lacto-ovo and lacto vegetarians can meet some of these needs with dairy foods (and eggs in the case of lacto-ovos), as they are rich in all of these nutrients. But I don't recommend that you increase your consumption of such foods to "make up for" not eating meat. The foods you should eat more of, because they are more nutrient-dense and nutrient-varied, are protein-rich plant foods including beans (especially soy, which contains all nine essential amino acids), nuts, seeds, and to a lesser extent whole grains. If you're a pure vegetarian or vegan these foods, as a group, should become your top nutrition priority.

Taking supplemental protein or amino acids in a post-run recovery drink will all but ensure that you get enough protein and make the most efficient possible use of the protein you get. Most such products use whey protein, which is derived from dairy, so if you're a pure vegetarian or vegan choose one that uses soy protein.

Good plant sources of vitamins B_2 and B_{12} include whole grains, green leafy vegetables, and nuts. These foods plus a variety of beans provide plenty of calcium as well. Beans, greens, whole grains, and fortified grains are also the best sources of iron, but the form of iron they contain is not easily absorbed. However, absorption of plant iron is greatly enhanced when it is consumed with vitamin C, which is abundant in tomatoes, citrus fruits and fruit juices, and broccoli, among other foods. To fill any gaps that may otherwise occur on any given day, take a daily multivitamin-multimineral supplement (as even nonvegetarians should do).

Throughout this book, I have continually come back to the theme that the same nutrition that enhances your overall well-being also boosts your running performance, and vice versa. In reading through this chapter, you will have seen that this rule holds across all subgroups within the running population. No matter which subgroup or -groups of runners you belong to, nourishing your general health will also benefit your running, and fueling your running better will enhance your general health. If you're overweight, trimming calories from your diet and getting the right calories at the right times will not only help you shed fat but will also help you run longer and stronger, which in turn will help you shed even more fat. If you're an older runner, making an effort to better fuel your recovery will turn back the clock on your running and at the same time make you feel and look younger.

One of the great qualities of running is the synergy between running and life. There's really no separation between running and the rest of life, between the runner and the human being. All the benefits you gain from running carry over into work, sleep, mood, and relationships, and a healthy, balanced lifestyle is the best possible foundation for running. If you could take only one lesson from this book, I hope it would be a clearer understanding of this synergy and the crucial role that nutrition has in it.

Eat well, run well, and live well!

INDEX

233